D1423741

Health Promotion Practice

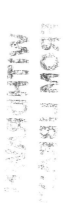

Understanding Public Health Series

Series editors: Nicki Thorogood and Rosalind Plowman, London School of Hygiene & Tropical Medicine (previous edition edited by Nick Black and Rosalind Raine)

Throughout the world, recognition of the importance of public health to sustainable, safe, and healthy societies is growing. The achievements of public health in nineteenth-century Europe were for much of the twentieth century overshadowed by advances in personal care, in particular in hospital care. Now, with the dawning of a new century, there is increasing understanding of the inevitable limits of individual health care and of the need to complement such services with effective public health strategies. Major improvements in people's health will come from controlling communicable diseases, eradicating environmental hazards, improving people's diets, and enhancing the availability and quality of effective health care. To achieve this, every country needs a cadre of knowledgeable public health practitioners with social, political, and organizational skills to lead and bring about changes at international, national, and local levels.

This is one of a series of books that provides a foundation for those wishing to join in and contribute to the twenty-first-century regeneration of public health, helping to put the concerns and perspectives of public health at the heart of policy-making and service provision. While each book stands alone, together they provide a comprehensive account of the three main aims of public health: protecting the public from environmental hazards, improving the health of the public, and ensuring high-quality health services are available to all. Some of the books focus on methods, others on key topics. They have been written by staff at the London School of Hygiene & Tropical Medicine with considerable experience of teaching public health to students from low-, middle-, and high-income countries. Much of the material has been developed and tested with postgraduate students both in face-to-face teaching and through distance learning.

The books are designed for self-directed learning. Each chapter has explicit learning objectives, key terms are highlighted, and the text contains many activities to enable the reader to test their own understanding of the ideas and material covered. Written in a clear and accessible style, the series will be essential reading for students taking postgraduate courses in public health and will also be of interest to public health practitioners and policy-makers.

Titles in the series

Analytical models for decision making: Colin Sanderson and Reinhold Gruen
Conflict and health: Natasha Howard, Egbert Sondorp and Annemarie Ter Veen (eds.)
Controlling communicable disease: Norman Noah
Economic analysis for management and policy: Stephen Jan, Lilani Kumaranayake, Jenny Roberts, Kara Hanson and Kate Archibald
Economic evaluation: Julia Fox-Rushby and John Cairns (eds.)
Environmental epidemiology: Paul Wilkinson (ed.)
Environmental health policy: Megan Landon and Tony Fletcher
Financial management in health services: Reinhold Gruen and Anne Howarth
Globalization and health, second edition: Johanna Hanefeld (ed.)
Health care evaluation: Sarah Smith, Don Sinclair, Rosalind Raine and Barnaby Reeves
Health promotion theory, second edition: Liza Cragg, Maggie Davies and Wendy Macdowall (eds.)
Introduction to epidemiology, second edition: Ilona Carneiro and Natasha Howard
Introduction to health economics, second edition: Lorna Guinness and Virginia Wiseman (eds.)
Issues in public health, second edition: Fiona Sim and Martin McKee (eds.)
Making health policy, second edition: Kent Buse, Nicholas Mays and Gill Walt
Managing health services: Nick Goodwin, Reinhold Gruen and Valerie Iles
Medical anthropology: Robert Pool and Wenzel Geissler
Principles of social research, second edition: Mary Alison Durand and Tracey Chantler (eds.)
Public health in history: Virginia Berridge, Martin Gorsky and Alex Mold
Sexual health: A public health perspective: Kay Wellings, Kirstin Mitchell and Martine Collumbien (eds.)
Understanding health services: Nick Black and Reinhold Gruen

Forthcoming titles

Environment, health and sustainable development, second edition: Emma Hutchinson and Sari Kovats

Health Promotion Practice

Second edition

Edited by Will Nutland and
Liza Cragg

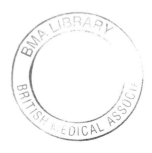

Mc
Graw
Hill
Education

Open University Press

Open University Press
McGraw-Hill Education
McGraw-Hill House
Shoppenhangers Road
Maidenhead
Berkshire
England
SL6 2QL

email: enquiries@openup.co.uk
world wide web: www.openup.co.uk

and Two Penn Plaza, New York, NY 10121-2289, USA

First published 2015

A catalogue record of this book is available from the British Library

ISBN-13: 978-0-33-526406-3 (pb)
ISBN-10: 0-33-526406-9 (pb)
eISBN: 978-0-33-526407-0

Library of Congress Cataloging-in-Publication Data
CIP data applied for

Typesetting and e-book compilations by
RefineCatch Limited, Bungay, Suffolk

Fictitious names of companies, products, people, characters and/or data that may be used herein (in case studies or in examples) are not intended to represent any real individual, company, product or event.

Contents

List of figures & tables

Figures

Tables

List of authors

JAMES CHAUVIN is a public health advocate and independent consultant. He was recently President of the World Federation of Public Health Associations and formerly Director of Policy at the Canadian Public Health Association.

LIZA CRAGG is a freelance consultant specializing in international health and teaches on several public health distance learning modules at the London School of Hygiene & Tropical Medicine.

MATT EGAN is a senior lecturer at the Department of Social and Environmental Health Research at the London School of Hygiene & Tropical Medicine.

ADAM FLETCHER is a senior lecturer in Social Science and Health at the Centre for the Development and Evaluation of Complex Interventions for Public Health Improvement, Cardiff University School of Social Sciences.

SIMON FORREST is a Senior Teaching Fellow at the School of Medicine and Health at Durham University.

ELAINE GARDNER is a freelance consultant specializing in food and nutrition and teaches on several public health distance learning modules at the London School of Hygiene & Tropical Medicine.

FORD HICKSON is a lecturer and course director for the Public Health MSc at the London School of Hygiene & Tropical Medicine.

LUCY LEE is a public health researcher specializing in global mental health and teaches on several modules at the London School of Hygiene & Tropical Medicine.

WILL NUTLAND is a Research Fellow and module organizer at the London School of Hygiene and Tropical Medicine. He was formerly head of health promotion at the UK's Terrence Higgins Trust and a public health strategist for the London Borough of Tower Hamlets.

MORTEN SKOVDAL is an Associate Professor of Global Health with the Section for Health Services Research, University of Copenhagen.

PAULA VALENTINE is a community mobilization and participation advisor with the Department of Programme Policy and Quality, Save the Children UK.

PETER WEATHERBURN is Director of Sigma Research and senior lecturer in Sexual Health & HIV at the London School of Hygiene & Tropical Medicine.

MEG WIGGINS is a senior research officer at the Social Science Research Unit, which is part of the Institute of Education, University of London.

HEATHER YEATMAN is Professor of Public and Population Health and head of the School of Health and Society at the University of Wollongong in New South Wales, Australia. She is also President of the Public Health Association of Australia.

Acknowledgements

This book is based on the distance learning module 'Principles and Practices of Health Promotion' and on the face-to-face modules 'Health Promotion Methods and Approaches' and 'Integrating Health Promotion', which are all taught as part of the Masters in Public Health at the London School of Hygiene & Tropical Medicine. These modules have evolved over several years under the influence of many staff. The editors are grateful to all these staff for providing learning materials and ideas that have been incorporated into this book. In particular, we would like to thank Chris Bonell, Adam Bourne, Maggie Davies, Elaine Gardner, Andy Guise, Wendy Macdowall, Ros Plowman, Nicki Thorogood, and Peter Weatherburn for their advice on the structure and content of this second edition. We would also like to thank students and teaching staff for providing useful feedback on the first edition of this book, which has been used to inform the development of this second edition. A number of case studies and examples for Chapter 3 are based upon work originally undertaken by Laura M. Duggan, Mar Estupiñan, Luis Guerra, Maiko Hirai, Stacey Mearns, Natalie Pedersen, Nadja Tariverdian, Felicity Williamson, and May Yoshikawa. We would like to thank the organizations and individuals who contributed information for case studies. In particular, thanks to the following for contributing case studies on therapeutic change: Florence Kerr-Corrêa, Professor of Psychiatry at Botucatu Medical School, Sao Paulo State University, Brazil; Rebecca Papas, Assistant Professor, Department of Psychiatry and Human Behavior at Brown University School of Public Health; and Kathleen Griffiths, Professor & Director of the National Institute for Mental Health Research at the Research School of Population Health at the Australian National University.

Open University Press and the London School of Hygiene & Tropical Medicine have made every effort to obtain permission from copyright holders to reproduce material in this book and to acknowledge these sources correctly. Any omissions brought to our attention will be remedied in future editions.

We would like to express our grateful thanks to the copyright holders for granting permission to reproduce material in this book from the following sources:

Craig, P., Dieppe, P., Macintyre, S., Michie, S., Nazareth, I. and Petticrew, M. (2008) *Developing and Evaluating Complex Interventions: New Guidance*. London: Medical Research Council. By permission of the Medical Research Council.

Dahlgren, G. and Whitehead, M. (1991) *Policies and Strategies to Promote Social Equity in Health*. Stockholm: Institute of Futures Studies. By permission of the World Health Organization.

Ross, A. and Chang, M. (2013) *Planning Healthier Places – Report from the Reuniting Health with Planning Project*. London: Town and Country Planning Association. By permission of the Town and Country Planning Association.

Rowe, F., Stewart, D. and Patterson, C. (2007) Promoting school connectedness through whole school approaches, *Health Education*, 107 (6): 524–42. By permission of Emerald Group Publishing.

Simmons, A., Mavoa, H.M. and Bell, A.C. (2009) Creating community action plans for obesity prevention using the ANGELO (Analysis Grid for Elements Linked to Obesity) Framework, *Health Promotion International*, 24 (4): 311–24. By permission of Oxford University Press.

Thakur, J.S., Bains, P., Kar, S.S., Wadhwa, S., Moirangthem, P., Kumar, R., Wadwalker, S. and Sharma, Y. (2012) Integrated healthy workplace model: an experience from North Indian industry, *Indian Journal of Occupational and Environmental Medicine*, 16 (3): 108–13. By permission of the *Indian Journal of Occupational and Environmental Medicine*.

World Health Organization (WHO) (2014) *Regional Activities: Approaches as Implemented in the WHO Regions*. Geneva: WHO. By permission of the World Health Organization [http://www.who.int/healthy_settings/regional/en/].

Overview of the book

Introduction

Health promotion is the process of enabling people to increase control over, and to improve, their health (WHO, 1986) and forms an important part of public health practice. Health promotion is not limited to addressing specific health problems or types of behaviour. It is also concerned with the range of social determinants that impact on health-related behaviour and health and well-being. Health promotion interventions may seek to prevent non-communicable diseases, communicable diseases, injury and violence, and mental illness. They may also seek to generate and emphasize social and personal resources to improve health and well-being.

The practice of health promotion is about much more than simply advising or persuading individuals to make lifestyle changes. Interventions can take place at different levels, including face-to-face contact with individuals, working with groups and communities, and strategic level work including policy development. Health promotion practice includes advocacy, community mobilization, policy development, advice, therapeutic support, and media information campaigns. This means that health promoters need a range of skills in, for example, needs assessment, partnership working, project management and evaluation, as well as a solid understanding of different methods used in health promotion interventions. This second edition of *Health Promotion Practice* describes these skills and methods and provides practical tools to help health promotion practitioners apply them. The content builds on *Health Promotion Theory*, another book in the Understanding Public Health series, which describes and explores the key principles and theory behind health promotion and its practice.

Why study health promotion practice?

As this book makes clear, health promotion practice is far from straightforward. It seeks to interact with individuals, groups, communities, and other stakeholders using a range of methods to influence change in what are often complex ways. Health promotion interventions must be carefully designed, planned, managed, and implemented in order to be effective and cost-efficient. The follow-up and evaluation of interventions also need careful consideration to ensure that, where possible, they generate learning that can contribute to developing the evidence base of what works. Furthermore, the methods used in health promotion practice are underpinned by theory and by evidence that indicate how they can be used most effectively. Unless public health practitioners understand this theory and evidence and use it to inform their practice, there is a risk that interventions could be ineffective or could even exacerbate the problems they seek to alleviate.

This book will guide you through the practical skills needed to plan, design, implement, and evaluate health promotion interventions. It will explain a wide range of methods that have been used to understand public health problems and develop effective health promotion responses to these problems. Throughout the book, the focus is firmly on assisting you to apply the skills and methods described in the implementation of health promotion activities in your own context.

Building on the first edition

This edition of *Health Promotion Practice* builds on the foundations of the first edition. Two major developments have shaped this second edition. First, as attention in health promotion practice globally realigns to focus on structural and environmental impacts on health, this edition gives greater emphasis and attention to upstream health promotion practice and interventions, including the development of healthy public policy and health advocacy. This is reflected both in the content of the book and its structure, with Section 2 introducing population-level interventions before moving on to community, sub-population, and then individual-focused health promotion interventions. Second, this edition gives greater emphasis to social media and web-based health promotion interventions, reflecting real-world changes in practice. Chapter 9 addresses some of the principles of the practice of social media and web-based media interventions and other chapters reflect developments in the use of web-focused technologies, such as online therapeutic methods, or the shift in the provision of information and advice methods using smart phones and apps.

The structure of the book

This book is structured in two sections. The first of these sections, comprising four chapters, provides practical guidance and tools for planning, delivering and evaluating health promotion. The second section, comprising a further nine chapters, looks at the range of different methods that are used in health promotion practice.

Each chapter follows the same format. A brief overview tells you about the contents, followed by learning objectives and the key terms you will encounter. There are several activities in each chapter, which are designed to help you practise applying the learning and tools introduced in the chapter and to test knowledge and understanding. Each activity is followed by feedback to enable you to check on your own understanding.

Section 1: Planning and delivering health promotion

The opening chapter of Section 1 explores some of the key concepts in health promotion practice. In doing so, it explains the complexity of issues with which health promotion engages, including the social determinants of health and how these impact on individual behaviour. It also discusses the many different stakeholders engaged in health promotion and the complex issues of acceptability and feasibility involved.

Chapter 2 addresses planning health promotion interventions. It provides an overview of some of the most common planning models and frameworks that have been developed for health promotion interventions. It then explains the key stages of planning a health promotion intervention and the practical steps involved.

Chapter 3 turns to implementing health promotion interventions. It stresses the importance of proper coordination and management in successful interventions and provides practical guidance on how these can be achieved. It also provides examples of tools that can be used in implementing health promotion interventions and critical factors for successful implementation.

The final chapter in Section 1 looks at evaluating and monitoring health promotion interventions. It explains why evaluation is important and introduces different types of evaluation often used in health promotion practice. It goes on to provide practical guidance on designing monitoring frameworks and carrying out evaluation.

Section 2: Methods used in health promotion

The second section of the book introduces the reader to different methods commonly used in health promotion to address societal, community, and individual determinants of health and illness, with each chapter dedicated to a different method. These chapters each give an overview of the method, describe how it can be most effectively used, provide tools for doing so, give examples, and suggest critical factors for success.

It should be stressed that a health promotion intervention or programme may use various combinations of methods to achieve their aims. So although necessarily arranged in discrete chapters, the reader should consider these methods as potentially complementary and to be used in combination rather than separately.

Chapter 5 is concerned with Healthy Public Policy (HPP) in health promotion practice. It describes how social policies beyond the health sector can be incorporated into public health strategies using HPP. It discusses key concepts underpinning HPP, and explores some of the challenges involved in its delivery.

Chapter 6 describes advocacy for health – a deliberate pro-activist process that uses strategic actions to influence others to address the underlying factors that affect human health. The chapter provides several frameworks to guide advocacy for health and practical case studies of how to undertake health advocacy.

Chapter 7 explains the concept of healthy settings, a concept that has moved from the more traditional view of settings as 'locations' to a broader idea of 'environments', and discusses some of the advantages and disadvantages of a healthy settings approach.

Chapter 8 describes the role of community mobilization in developing healthy communities. It highlights various tools and methods that can be used to mobilize communities and illustrates how these can be applied in practice through a discussion of 'real-world' community mobilization projects.

Chapter 9 explains a broad range of media-focused methods, including mass media, social media, and social marketing. It emphasizes the growing importance of social media in health promotion practices and reflects the growing use of interactive media methods of health promotion.

Chapter 10 explains how peer education is used as a method of health promotion. It describes some of the theories about health-related behaviour and considers some of the challenges faced by policy-makers and practitioners in planning and implementing peer education.

Chapter 11 looks at therapeutic change methods used in health promotion, including cognitive behavioural therapy, motivational interviewing, and online methods of delivery. It explores the theoretical models that underpin these methods and provides case studies to illustrate how they are used in practice.

Chapter 12 explores information and advice methods, including common methods used in health promotion such as outreach and detached work; theatre and performance; and audio and visual methods. It explores how information and advice methods are changing with new media technologies.

The final chapter discusses how health promotion interventions and programmes combine different methods in order to address the determinants of health *at multiple levels* at the same time. It explains how combining multiple methods amplifies the complexity of delivery and explores these practical challenges by presenting real-life case studies from a range of contexts and settings.

Brief explanation of terminology

There are a number of terms that are used in different ways by different organizations involved in health promotion and public health. Different terms are often used interchangeably and this can be frustrating for those studying health promotion. However, in real-life health promotion practice such uniformity of language use often does not exist and to suggest it does by providing rigid definitions would be misleading. For the sake of clarity, the key terms that are often confused and how they are used within this book are given below.

- *Health promotion intervention*: a purposeful activity for a defined group using finite resources to prevent disease and/or promote positive health.
- *Health promotion project*: often used interchangeably with *health promotion intervention*. In this book, *health promotion intervention* is generally used.
- *Health promotion programme*: used in this book to refer to a number of health promotion interventions that share the same overarching aim(s). In real life, *programme* is sometimes used interchangeably with *project*.
- *Intervention approach*: sometimes used to describe the way an intervention is carried out, for example a community development approach. Sometimes used interchangeably with *intervention method*. In this book, *intervention method* is used and where the word *approach* is used, it has no technical meaning.
- *Intervention method*: used in this book to describe how an intervention will achieve its aim(s), for example mass media, information and advice, and therapeutic methods.
- *Intervention type*: sometimes used to categorize different methods, for example behavioural, educational or psychological intervention types. Sometimes used interchangeably with *intervention method*. In this book, *intervention method* is used and where the word *type* is used, it has no technical meaning.

The use of the terms *health promotion* and *public health* can also be confusing. In this book, *health promotion* is used in accordance with the WHO definition to mean the process of enabling people to increase control over and to improve their health. *Health promotion* is a key element of the broader discipline of *public health,* which also includes activities generally considered to be outside the scope of health promotion, such as disease surveillance, preparing for potential health emergencies, and managing vaccination programmes. However, there is no universally accepted way of defining exactly which activities do and do not fall within health promotion, as opposed to public health. Often the issues with which health promotion engages are referred to as public health concerns or priorities. In addition, some organizations use the term public health rather than health promotion. Therefore, readers are encouraged to accept the fluidity of these terms.

Each chapter also includes a list of key terms and their definitions in its opening paragraphs. These key terms are brought together in a glossary at the end of the book.

Reference

World Health Organization (WHO) (1986) *Ottawa Charter for Health Promotion.* Geneva: WHO [http://www.who.int/healthpromotion/conferences/previous/ottawa/en/; accessed 18 October 2012].

SECTION 1

Planning and delivering health promotion

Concepts in health promotion 1

Ford Hickson

Overview

This first chapter introduces the concept of health promotion need. As the chapter explains, states of health and illness have multiple causes that arise through complex chains of causes and effects involving many actors. The chapter goes on to explore the key features of a health promotion intervention and to introduce the concept of programmes of health promotion interventions. Because of the complexity involved, the chapter proposes that health promotion frequently requires a programmatic approach, rather than a one-off, single intervention. Finally, the chapter identifies the different actors responsible for health promotion and outlines the role each may have in a health promotion programme.

Learning objectives

After reading this chapter, you will be able to:

- distinguish between an activity and an intervention
- describe the five key dimensions of an intervention
- distinguish between an intervention and a programme
- understand the range of actors responsible for health promotion needs of a population

Key terms

Health-related needs: Attributes people need to have to be able to control their health-related behaviour: knowledge and awareness; access to resources; interpersonal skills and physical motor skills; and bodily autonomy.

Intervention: Purposeful activity using finite resources that is carried out with the aim of changing something specific for a defined group of people.

Programme: A number of interlinked interventions addressing a common health issue or problem (or a target group).

Introduction

States of health and disease are influenced by a wide range of factors. The Lalonde Report (1974), which was instrumental in the foundation of health promotion as a discipline, grouped these influences into four broad categories: biology, lifestyle, environment, and health care. Within each of these categories there are multiple and potentially diverse factors that influence health.

For example, the incidence of breast cancer is known to be affected by biological factors including genetic inheritance and age; lifestyle factors including exercise and alcohol consumption; and health care factors including preventative drugs such as tamoxifen and raloxifene, or surgical prevention though mastectomy. The environmental factors that may contribute to breast cancer are less well understood. However, breast cancer incidence is higher in industrialized countries and the majority of women who develop breast cancer have no recognized genetic or lifestyle risk factor. This suggests there may be unrecognized links to the environment.

Understanding the causes of health and disease is essential for taking action to influence them. However, the contribution of different factors to health and disease states is often controversial. One controversy concerns whether a specific factor makes any contribution at all, or how important it is relative to other factors. Controversy is often related to the value people place on the factor itself and what its identification as a risk factor for disease suggests should be done about it.

Understanding health needs

Health needs are the things that give us control over the factors that influence our health. For example, the needs related to eating a healthy diet might include knowledge about different foods and their nutritional value, access to fresh fruit and vegetables, an ability to prepare them for consumption, and the time and facilities to do so. Health needs can be identified by asking individuals themselves, known as expressed needs, and/or by experts identifying them on the basis of logic or research, known as normative needs.

The needs related to doing something may be different from the needs related to changing from not doing it, to doing it. So, for example, changing from an unhealthy to a healthy diet may also require knowledge of what is healthy or unhealthy and social approval for healthy eating. Since health promotion interventions are usually intended to bring about change, they need to attend to both the needs required for a behaviour and the needs required to change towards that behaviour.

The extent to which health needs are met is dictated by the actions of all of those around us, including policy-makers, services, and communities. Policy-makers include legislators in central and local governments as well as strategic decision-makers in other organizations, and it is policy-makers – rather than people delivering services – who usually determine which and how services are delivered. The actions of people in education, health, and social services may not be fully aligned with what policy-makers intend, and services may vary depending on whom they are delivered to and thus the quality of services may also vary enormously. Everyone is a member of one or more communities, and many people's health needs are met through families, friends, and neighbours. Businesses (other than health, education, and social services) can also be thought of as part of the community, and the nature and distribution of shops and services greatly influences whether people have control over their own health.

Activity 1.1

This activity encourages you to reflect on factors that influence health. Think about the following questions:

1   What does it mean to be healthy?
2   What factors help people to be healthy and stay healthy?
3   What are some of the causes of ill health?
4   What are the causes of these causes of ill health?

Feedback

In answer to the first question, you might have concluded that being healthy means not being ill or in pain. But health is more than this. The World Health Organization's definition of health is 'not merely the absence of disease but a state of complete physical, mental and social well-being'. In response to the second question, your answer may have included factors such as having access to healthy food, clean water, health care, appropriate housing and sanitation. In addition to these basic needs, you might have included lifestyle factors such as taking exercise, getting rest, being relaxed and free from stress. Moving on to question 3, lacking these basic things causes ill health but ill health can also be caused by lifestyle factors such as unhealthy eating, smoking or lack of exercise. In response to question 4, your answer should reflect that the causes of the causes of ill health also include poverty, economic and social inequality, weak education, lack of employment opportunities or hazardous working conditions, inadequate access to health care or poor quality health care, poor quality physical environment, pollution, and lack of support networks.

What is a health promotion intervention?

An intervention is any purposeful and planned activity, carried out in a specific place, with the intention of bringing about some kind of change in a specific person or group of people. Without a purpose and a plan, an activity should not be considered an intervention. The purpose of a health promotion intervention is to address the requirements for action that is to meet the needs of a specific person or group of people. These needs depend on the health- or illness-related behaviour they are trying to change. Chapter 2 provides a more detailed explanation of needs assessment.

Thus, for an activity to be considered an intervention, we must specify the *aims* of the activity, their setting, and the intended target. How the intervention will achieve its aims are the *objectives*. The *resources* required to carry out the intervention must also be described. The place the activities take place in is the *setting or site* for the intervention. The person or people the intervener intends to change things for can be called the *target*.

These, then, are the five essential dimensions of any intervention: aims, setting, target, objectives, and resources. A coherent intervention description is one in which there is congruence between the dimensions, such that the aim is achievable with the objectives (not, for example, developing a motor skill by reading a leaflet), the target can be encountered in the setting (not, for example, people with lower levels of education in a university), and the objectives are feasible in the setting and within the resources available.

This chapter now discusses definitions, theoretical concepts, and areas of contention of each of these dimensions in turn, while Chapter 2 goes on to provide practical guidance on how they should be addressed in the process of planning an intervention.

Intervention aims

The aims of an intervention, how they are described, and how far they extend are determined by the purpose of the intervention. There is an ongoing debate as to the purpose of health promotion interventions, and consequently the meaning of their success. Broadly speaking there are two camps: those who hold that the meaning of success is that people have control over their own health (whether or not they pursue a healthy option) and those who hold that the meaning of success is that people behave in a way prescribed by the intervener (whether or not people have the choice of doing so or are happy about it). In the first case, the purpose of health promotion intervention is to increase the control people have over their own health, in the second case, the purpose is to encourage people to adopt behaviours that the intervener considers healthy.

According to the definition of the Ottawa Charter (WHO, 1986), in health promotion the purpose of an intervention is to meet health needs. That is, to increase the control the target has over the factors influencing their health. The health promoter does not have the right to impose change on the target and it is the target who decides the ideal behavioural outcome. That people make a specific decision (or act in a specific way) is not the goal but rather that they have the knowledge, skills, resources, and opportunities to take the action they choose, and they understand the consequences of those actions for their health, or the health and well-being of others. Once those needs are met, the health promoter's job is done.

The behaviour changer, on the other hand, assumes the right to say what the best behavioural outcome is. However, they must still operate through needs, although they are more likely to be defined normatively and may include limiting opportunities to take risks as well as meeting needs for taking precaution (for example, supplying resources). The behaviour changer's job is not done until the population conforms to their prescribed behaviour(s).

Two interventions that seek to change the same behaviour may well have different aims because they bring about change through meeting different needs. For example, a condom distribution scheme (through access to a material resource) and a TV advert (through developing social norms about using condoms) both might seek to increase condom use.

Intervention targets

The description for the target of an intervention can include both the characteristics of its *potential* audience (all the people who may potentially benefit) as well as indicating *how many* of the potential audience it is hoped will be reached (either as a proportion of the potential audience or a specific number of people).

When the intervention is encountered directly by the population of concern, the target group should be defined to maximize the impact of the intervention. This is usually the group of people who are most in need of what the intervention has to offer. A description of the target group is therefore a surrogate marker for either the health concern at issue or the specific needs the intervention addresses. For example, an intervention concerned with increasing exercise should have as its target group those people less likely to exercise. If the intervention specifically increases knowledge of a sports facility, the target should be those less likely to already know about it.

The specified target group should be as comprehensive as possible. So, for example, 'young people' does not mean 'young heterosexual people' unless it explicitly says so. An intervention whose target is simply 'young people' should be expected to be of equal benefit to gay and lesbian, bisexual and heterosexual young people, young people from ethnic minorities as well as the ethnic majority, disabled young people as well as able-bodied young people, and so on. It should also be expected to benefit young men as well as young women, unless specified otherwise.

The profile of people whose needs are intended to change as a result of intervention activities should include a consideration of gender, age, ethnicity, sexuality, disability, class/occupation/education, area of residence, as well as other characteristics. Characteristics of the population not specified indicate that the intervener considers that characteristic to be unimportant for health inequalities, the behaviour of concern, and the specific needs the intervention is intended to address.

Because health is the outcome of the actions of many different people along the chain of causation, health promotion interventions may be targeted at, for example, government ministers and other policy-makers, newspaper editors, service commissioners and service providers, as well as directed at the population of concern. If the intervention is targeted at any of these people, the intervention description should be as precise as possible about who these people are. In this case, the potential target audience is usually much smaller than the potential target audience among the general public.

✎ Activity 1.2

Study the specified target group for an intervention (either a health promoter's description or in an evaluation report). Does it include information about where the intended target group live, their sex, age, ethnicity, disability, occupation or education? What other characteristics are mentioned (exclude those based on where the intervention occurs or what the aim of the intervention is)? Considering these seven characteristics (residence, sex, age, ethnicity, sexuality, disability, education/occupation level), which sub-groups do you think are most likely to encounter the intervention?

Feedback

There is no health concern that is equally distributed across all characteristics of the population. No intervention is encountered by all members of its potential target group and all interventions have target group biases. For example, social media interventions are disproportionately seen by some sections of their target group more than others, and places on skills courses are taken more frequently by some groups. The potential target group for an intervention should specify, where relevant, the desirable biases in who gets the intervention. For example, is the intervention intended to be encountered equally by those with no educational qualifications as by those with university education? If not, which sub-groups should be served more than others?

Intervention settings and sites

The setting for an intervention is the type of context within which the intervention activities take place. An intervention site is a specific geographic location.

The settings in which intervention activities take place determine who encounters and therefore benefits from them. All intervention activities must take place somewhere and the place they occur in is a key determinant of both their feasibility and the profile of the people who encounter them. Although no specific activities can be done everywhere, there are few places where no health promotion activities could be conducted. This means the potential range of settings for health promotion interventions is enormous. Common settings for health promotion interventions include: on-line and off-line media (social networks, press, radio, television); the street; businesses (pubs, clubs, restaurants); schools; community and religious centres (churches, mosques, synagogues, temples); service centres (hospitals, clinics, organizational bases); care homes; prisons; and personal homes. In addition, interventions targeted at the needs for action of, for example, policy-makers and service providers can occur through professional networks.

Many of the above settings are places where people are present for some reason other than health promotion activities. Activities in these settings do not usually require a recruitment element (the people are already there). Interventions occurring in places where people are required to attend (where the targets for the intervention have to come to the intervener) usually require additional promotion, which can take the form of a different intervention. Many settings in which an intervention itself may not be feasible may nevertheless be suitable for recruitment interventions.

Intervention objectives

Generally, aims are where you want to be and objectives are what you do to get there. What constitutes an objective depends on where an aim is pitched. For example, if our aim is to reduce new sexually acquired HIV infections, our objective could be to reduce sexual HIV exposures. Subsequently, if our aim is to reduce sexual HIV exposures, our objectives could be to increase knowledge, social norms for condom use, condom use skills, access to condoms, and so on. Then, if our aim is to increase knowledge, our objectives could be to organize facilitated discussion groups and recruitment to them.

At the most immediate level, objectives are the things you do that constitute the intervention. This is the first level at which objectives can be specified and it is what is meant when we refer to intervention objectives. Objectives include the sequence of events as well as the methods and approaches being used. The different methods and approaches commonly used in health promotion to address individual, community, and social determinants of health and illness are covered in Section 2 of the book. There is no simple divide between effective and ineffective methods; rather, different methods are more or less effective at achieving different aims with different groups in different settings.

Note that the objectives include both what the target group does as well as what the intervener does. An intervention cannot be said to have occurred if a leaflet is put in a rack but no one ever picks it up and reads it. It is the act of reading that completes the objectives of the intervention.

Small media such as leaflets and postcards require a distribution mechanism to get them into people's hands. So, for example, a leaflet is not in itself an intervention. Similarly, some objectives are incomplete without a front-end. Recruitment is often an essential element of an intervention and should be included in the description of the activities. The objectives for an outreach session, for example, could include: arrange with the bar owner/manager to visit and work the site; attend the site; approach and engage people in the target group; listen and talk to establish and address unmet needs; and distribute leaflets and condoms.

Intervention resources

A description of an intervention should include the resources required to carry out the intervention activities. While resources can be expressed financially, there may also be some resources that cannot be purchased by the health promoter. So, for example, a safer sex outreach session in a community setting, such as a bar or club, requires: trained outreach workers, resources to distribute (leaflets, condoms), and a bar or club in which to carry out the work.

Qualities of interventions

Evaluation usually asks questions about the qualities or performance of an intervention. Evaluation is discussed in more detail in Chapter 4. However, it is worth stressing that without an intervention plan, we cannot evaluate an intervention. If we describe the aims and targets, setting and activities of an intervention, we can say something about its qualities and whether it was successful. Qualities of health promotion interventions that are often evaluated include:

- **Feasibility** refers to whether or not the activities can be done in the setting with the available resources. Activities feasible in in some settings will not be feasible in others.
- **Acceptability** is what both the intervener but especially the target thinks about the activities and their outcomes, whether they like or dislike (or feel neutral towards) them. The extent to which it is important that the target actually enjoys the activities of health promotion is a value held by some interveners and not others.
- **Coverage and access** are measures of penetration into the potential target audience (how many or what proportion encountered the activities) and also the biases in encountering the interventions. These qualities can only be described if we have described a target group. If we are uninterested in social equality, we can ignore the target group and just count all people encountered, but this is likely to undermine the impact of our activities because it ignores need.
- **Efficacy and effectiveness** both refer to whether or not the intervention brings about the intended aim for the target group. The distinction between them is taken from clinical interventions and is based on the impact a drug or procedure has in clinical trials and 'ideal conditions' (its efficacy) and the impact it has in real-life practice (its effectiveness). In social and educational interventions, the distinction between the efficacy and effectiveness of interventions is less clear, as few such interventions can be delivered in laboratory conditions. Most health promotion interventions are studied in real life settings, even in evaluation designs that aspire to be trials.
- **Cost and cost-effectiveness** refer to the unit price of the intervention, either the entire intervention, a unit of output (cost per so many activities), or a unit of outcome (cost per so much change in needs, behaviours or morbidities in a particular target group). It is important to attend to the target group when considering cost-effectiveness, as the same change may be easier (or cheaper) to bring about in some groups than others.

🖉 **Activity 1.3**

What success looks like for a health promotion intervention with an individual is likely to be different to what success looks like for a health promotion programme with a population. Considering an example of a health promotion topic area you are familiar with, try to establish how the success of an intervention in that topic area with an individual might look different to success with a population of people. Why might that be?

Feedback

There is a distinction to be made between success for health promotion interventions with individuals and success for populations. A health promotion intervention with an individual should take account of the individual's values and preferences, and it is the individual him or herself who determines the desired outcome of the intervention. For example, in the context of safer sex, this may be abstaining from sex, having non-penetrative sex, using condoms or using pre-exposure prophylaxis. If the individual was formerly having no sex because they were too scared to do so, but decides, following an education and skills intervention, to start having intercourse with condoms, that individual's risk has in fact increased rather than decreased. However, for the individual the intervention was a success because they have more control over their choices. A safer sex programme for a population, on the other hand, might be judged a success only if there was an overall health gain in the population, with more people moving towards less risk than people moving towards risk. This health gain could also be people being happier with their sex lives.

What counts as a programme?

The term 'programme' is sometimes used for the scaling up of a single type of intervention to a large number of people (for example, provision of vaccination across a whole population might be termed a vaccination programme). However, it is more commonly used to refer to a collection of interventions that are individually intended to bring about diverse changes in a variety of targets, but which share a common overarching aim(s). The aim may be very narrow (for example, to reduce HIV transmissions) or it may be very broad (for example, to meet the expressed health needs of a village). Programmes are sometimes also called multi-level because they seek to achieve change at multiple levels, such as the individual, community, and policy levels. This is discussed further in Chapter 13. They are also sometimes known as complex interventions. Interventions may be complex because they:

- consist of diverse activities in a range of settings that interact with each other (for example, advertising, community discussion, advice sessions);
- tailor activities to individual targets or sub-groups of the target group (for example, screening and allocation of resources, writing letters to individuals);
- aim to influence a range of behaviours and/or health outcomes in a population of concern (for example, chlamydia screening, sexual negotiation skills *and* appropriate contraceptive use among teenage females), and therefore aim to influence a range of needs;

- have diverse target groups who are at different stages of change (for example, pre-contemplation, preparation, maintenance), and therefore again must influence a range of needs;
- have diverse targets with varying relationships to the population of concern (for example, policy-makers, business owners, and the population of concern itself).

Who is responsible for the health promotion needs of a population?

How health needs are defined is a political action because it dictates, to some extent, who is responsible for responding to them and what interventions are required. For example, limiting healthy eating needs to 'knowledge' means that only information interventions are required and that this can be supplied by health educators. If we recognize that access to cheap fruit and vegetables, adequate food preparation facilities, and skills are also healthy eating needs, then trading standards, housing and adult education colleges may also need to be involved. Unemployment and the local business economy become key in a population's healthy eating habits, rather than simply whether people know 'the healthy eating rules'.

There are numerous health issues unequally distributed between and within countries. The size and nature of responses to health issues varies, both over time and across populations. Whether a health issue is responded to is often related to who is being affected by it. Health issues that are limited to or mainly affect already marginalized groups (for example, tuberculosis, HIV, sickle cell anaemia) are less likely to garner public and political support for action than are those that affect either the 'general population' or mainstream groups such as children. This means that impacting on health issues affecting 'unpopular' groups may require changing the political context in which the health promotion intervention is carried out.

Policy-makers and commissioners, service providers, businesses and other community members share a need for collective, coherent, and coordinated responses to health issues. With an increase in the numbers and types of actors engaged in the response to health issues, there is a concomitant need for partnerships, referrals, and exchange of learning. These needs also require to be addressed and are appropriate aims for health promotion interventions.

A typology of health promotion action: building a programme

As many stakeholders are involved in addressing or undermining health promotion needs, health promotion interventions can involve many groups of people in addition to the group whose behaviour we are concerned with. Health promotion is affected by various areas of policy, numerous services, and the common conduct of much of the population. Many of these actions make health-related needs worse, especially with regards to the needs of socially unpopular groups, such as sexual minorities, migrants, drug users, smokers or prisoners. Health promotion resources may need to be spent on removing obstacles or preventing stigma, as well as on building knowledge or skills.

In very broad terms it is useful to think about three major constituencies of actors in the health-promoting fields, each of which may be instigator, intervener or target of an intervention. These are: community members, including business owners; policy-makers and resource allocators; and education, health, and social services personnel. Each of these constituencies is diverse and may target itself (community members may act on other businesses, for example, or politicians lobby other politicians).

Any action that contributes towards meeting health-related needs for any target group can be viewed as a valid health promotion activity. This means it is possible to have interventions that benefit a population of concern without them directly encountering the intervention. Health promotion programmes often seek to increase health promotion activity in others, such as services, businesses, and community members. They may also aim to reduce the health-damaging effects of actions by these constituencies.

All the potential actors themselves have needs for action that can be met by other actors. For example, service providers have skills and knowledge needs that can be met through training by education services, and politicians need awareness of their constituents' concerns that can be met through lobbying by community members. Action must arise from somewhere in order for a health situation to change.

Table 1.1 outlines the range of elements that might be included in a national response to a health issue. The specific examples relate to the HIV epidemic among men who have

Table 1.1 Elements that might be included in a national response to a health issue

Actors	Aim and target of intervention	Examples of interventions in a national HIV prevention programme
Policy-makers, resource allocators, and researchers	The needs of policy-makers, resource allocators, and researchers	• National evidence base • Public funds
	The needs of education, health, and social service providers	• Prevention strategies/plans • Development of HIV vaccines and microbicides
	The needs of community members	• Leadership against stigma and discrimination
	The health-related needs of the population of concern	• Social equality and justice legislation
Education, health, and social service providers	The needs of policy-makers, resource allocators, and researchers	• Professional associations and representation in policy-making, research, and resource allocation
	The needs of education, health, and social service providers	• Training and professional development • National and local collaborative planning fora
	The needs of community members	• Community development
	The health-related needs of the population of concern	• Equitable generic education, health, and social services: – HIV/STI testing – HIV/STI treatment – Education and counselling – Condoms and lubricants
Community members	The needs of policy-makers, resource allocators, and researchers	• Political action and lobbying
	The needs of education, health, and social service providers	• Public involvement in service planning
	The needs of community members	• Voluntary associations and community mobilization
	The health-related needs of the population of concern	• Peer education

sex with men, but the categories of intervention are applicable to all health issues. The typology gives us twelve different types of intervention in three groups of four. Usually, health promoters will only consider interventions they themselves do, but they also have a major role in facilitating the action of others.

Summary of learning points

This chapter has introduced important concepts concerned with planning and delivering health promotion interventions. It has described why, for an activity to be considered an intervention, it must specify, in advance, its intended target and aim, as well as the proposed activities and settings. As the needs associated with a health issue in a population are usually varied, the interventions required to address it also need to be varied. Groups of interventions addressing a common health issue or problem are often described as a programme. The target of a health promotion intervention need not be the population whose behaviour is the primary concern, but can be other actors who impact on that population (such as policy-makers, service providers, or community members and businesses). The following chapters in Section 1 of the book discuss how to plan and evaluate health promotion interventions and programmes. Chapter 13 builds on the concept of programmatic health promotion by providing case studies of multi-level health promotion interventions and the challenges in developing and evaluating these.

References

Lalonde, M. (1974) *A New Perspective on the Health of Canadians: A Working Document*. Ottawa: Government of Canada [reprinted 1981: http://www.phac-aspc.gc.ca/ph-sp/pdf/perspect-eng.pdf].

World Health Organization (WHO) (1986) *The Ottawa Charter for Health Promotion* [http://www.who.int/health-promotion/conferences/previous/ottawa/en/; accessed 10 September 2014].

Further reading

Bartholomew, L.K., Parcel, G.S., Kok, G., Gottlieb, N.H. and Fernandez, M.E. (2011) *Planning Health Promotion Programs: An Intervention Mapping Approach*, 3rd edn. Hoboken, NJ: Wiley.

Medical Research Council (2011) *Developing and Evaluating Complex Interventions: New Guidance* [www.mrc.ac.uk/complexinterventionsguidance; accessed 10 September 2014].

2 Planning health promotion interventions

Liza Cragg, Will Nutland and Ford Hickson

Overview

Health promotion interventions need to be carefully planned in order to be effective. This chapter describes the different tasks involved in planning an intervention and how to approach these tasks. The chapter also explores several models that have been developed to guide the planning of health promotion interventions. It discusses the importance of articulating the information gathered through the planning process in a single document and how to go about doing this. Chapter 3 goes on to explore how to implement and complete health promotion interventions.

Learning objectives

After reading this chapter, you will be able to:

- describe the key tasks involved in planning health promotion interventions
- understand how to go about undertaking these tasks
- employ several models used to undertake health promotion planning

Key terms

Aim: A broad statement of what will change as a result of an intervention.

Method: How an intervention will achieve its aim(s), for example through the use of mass media, peer education or community mobilization.

Objectives: Specific, concrete statements of what the intervention needs to achieve in order to reach its aim.

Plan: A document produced as a result of the process of planning the intervention which establishes the scope, aims, setting, target group, objectives, methods, and activities.

Introduction: Why is planning important and what is involved?

There are several reasons why planning is essential for health promotion interventions to be effective. First, health promotion involves an ethical imperative to be explicit about the assumptions, values, and principles on which it is based. This imperative can only be met if there is a clear rationale for an intervention and a transparent process for its development and implementation.

Second, planning the intervention involves defining and articulating the rationale behind it. This includes specifying the problem being addressed, the target group, the proposed method, what the intervention is trying to change, the theory of change being used, and the existing evidence that this will work. The process of describing this rationale will help identify any problems with the intervention design before resources and time are committed.

Third, as discussed in Chapter 1, effective health promotion often requires a multi-level or programmatic approach. This means that a health promotion programme will involve the interaction and interdependence of several interventions. Unless each of these is well managed, the success of the other interventions and the programme as a whole could be jeopardized.

Fourth, health promotion requires the involvement of many different participants and stakeholders. On a practical level, the success of the intervention will require input from individuals and agencies with relevant expertise and experience at the planning stage and throughout implementation. On an ethical level, potential users and beneficiaries of an intervention should be involved in decision-making. For this involvement to be meaningful it needs to be planned and managed to ensure the right people and agencies are involved at the right time.

Fifth, health promotion involves the investment of substantial sums of public money. Health promotion agencies must ensure that this funding is used for the purposes for which it was allocated, that value for money is obtained, and that money is properly accounted for. This requires proper planning of how resources will be used.

Sixth, having a clear plan allows other health promoters to transfer and scale-up interventions in other settings or with other target groups. Without a clear plan, it is not possible to replicate a successful intervention.

Finally, the intervention needs to be monitored and evaluated. The increased emphasis on evidence-based practice within health promotion means that it is important to show if an intervention met its aims and objectives. This also means the aims and objectives of an intervention need to be defined from the start. It is not possible to judge the success of an intervention if you cannot say definitively what it intended to achieve (and how it intended to achieve it).

The key tasks that are involved in planning an intervention are:

- Defining the need for the intervention;
- Identifying and engaging stakeholders;
- Defining aims and objectives;
- Selecting intervention methods;
- Reviewing the evidence of the effectiveness of the proposed method;
- Defining intended outcomes and outputs;
- Identifying the required resources;
- Identifying risks and assumptions;
- Planning for monitoring and evaluation;
- Planning for the project completion or scale-up;
- Developing a plan – the document that brings together information from all the above tasks.

These tasks will be outlined in turn later in the chapter.

While some of these tasks follow on from each other, others need to be carried out simultaneously or may need to be revisited as the plan evolves. In addition, the process of planning will need to be adapted to each intervention and will depend on different factors, including the size and complexity of the intervention, the capacity of the implementing agencies, the amount of funding available, the number of different stakeholders, and the impetus for developing the intervention. This means there is not necessarily a 'one-size-fits-all' model for planning health promotion interventions.

 Activity 2.1

Many planning models identify a linear or circular stage process, usually with the identification of needs at the start. However, in practice planning does not always occur in such a neat step-by-step format. Can you think of reasons why and examples of why planning might start at different stages?

Feedback

There are many reasons why it may not be possible to follow the stages for planning interventions in order, starting with establishing need. These include:

- The commissioner or funders may have already identified problems or needs that proposed interventions should address, for example in response to a new government policy.
- The commissioner or funders may have already specified the size and focus of an intervention. This could mean the resources/budget (for example, 1m is available) or the setting (for example, prisons, schools or entertainment venues) has been dictated.
- The commissioner or funders may have specified which method interventions should use, for example an existing type of intervention or a new innovative one.
- An organization or individual may instigate an intervention after having already identified what needs to be addressed. For example, a community group campaigning for traffic calming.

The reality is that many planning processes do not have as their first step the establishment of need. However, even if the need for the intervention has already been specified, it is important to describe and quantify this need in the plan for the intervention.

Health promotion planning models

A range of models has been developed to help practitioners conceptualize and undertake the planning of health promotion interventions. Such models usually break down the planning process into a number of interdependent tasks. While they share many features and propose similar planning tasks, they often use different terminology and conceptualize the interrelationships between tasks differently. Some of the most commonly used models are described briefly below.

PRECEDE-PROCEED

Proposed by Green and Kreuter (2005), the PRECEDE-PROCEED model distinguishes between the planning and the implementation stages of intervention. PRECEDE is an acronym used to describe the planning and developmental stages of the model. These are: **P**redisposing, **R**einforcing, and **E**nabling **C**onstructs in **E**cological **D**iagnosis and **E**valuation. PROCEED is an acronym used to describe the implementation of strategies and evaluation stages. These are: **P**olicy, **R**egulatory, and **O**rganizational **C**onstructs in **E**ducational and **E**nvironmental **D**evelopment.

The PRECEDE-PROCEED model stresses that, for the intervention to be effective, the determinants of health behaviour must be identified before the intervention is designed. In doing so, it distinguishes between three categories of factors that contribute to health behaviour:

1 Predisposing factors, which motivate an individual or group to take action, such as knowledge, beliefs, attitudes, values, and cultural norms;
2 Enabling factors, representing personal skills and available resources needed to perform a behaviour; and
3 Reinforcing factors, providing incentives for health behaviours and outcomes to be maintained.

PABCAR

The PABCAR model is a practical tool for health programme planning developed by Maycock *et al.* (2001). PABCAR is an acronym of the five key steps the model proposes. These are:

1 **P**roblem identification: What is the problem? What is its significance for the community?
2 **A**menable to change: Can you change the factors that cause the problem? How do you know?
3 **B**enefits and **C**osts: What are the social, ethical, and economic costs and benefits of intervening? The benefits should generally outweigh the costs.
4 **A**cceptability: Will the target group welcome the intervention or, at least, not oppose it?
5 **R**ecommendations for action and monitoring.

Framework for Public Health Practice

The Planning Framework for Public Health Practice (NPHP, 2000) is a tool to improve planning and management in public health, drawing from the common elements in existing planning processes in public health to effect rigour and consistency in intervention planning. The framework entails six steps:

• Identify the determinants of the health problem, the context in which they operate, and the population groups affected;
• Assess the risks and benefits posed by each determinant to identify what should be addressed;
• Identify intervention options and appraise them, including the level of evidence for their effectiveness;
• Decide the portfolio of interventions that can address the problem;
• Implement the portfolio;
• Evaluate the portfolio.

ASTOR

ASTOR is a way of remembering five dimensions that need to be defined as part of planning all health promotion interventions. These dimensions are **A**im, **S**etting, **T**arget, **O**bjectives, and **R**esources. An intervention can be planned starting with any of the five dimensions. Questions that help define these dimensions, using different starting points, include:

Start with an aim/need
   Who has the aim/need poorly met?
      Where can they be encountered?
         What activities that reduce the need can be done there?
            What resources are required?

Start with a target group
   What needs do they have unmet?
      Where can they be encountered?
         What activities that reduce the need can be done there?
            What resources are required?

Start with some resources
   Whose needs do you want to address?
      What needs/aims do they have poorly met?
         Where can they be encountered?
            What can be done there within the resources that will address unmet needs?

Start with a setting
   What activities can be done there?
      Who can be encountered there?
         What unmet needs do they have that can be addressed with feasible activities?
            What resources are required?

Start with objectives/tools
   What resources are required?
      Where can the objectives be done?
         Who can be encountered there?
            What needs that can be addressed by the available tools do the target have unmet?

The practical steps in planning an intervention

Defining the need for the intervention

It is important to understand health needs in order to design and implement a relevant and effective health promotion intervention. It is also essential to be clear about these needs in order to explain the rationale for the intervention. Assessing health needs is not straightforward, as it involves unpicking complex concepts such as 'health', 'illness' or 'need' and asking: What is health, what are the causes of health and illness, and what is need in this context? These concepts are discussed briefly here.

'Health' is a positive concept defined by the World Health Organization as 'a state of complete physical, mental and social well-being and not merely the absence of disease or infirmity' (WHO, 1948). Health and well-being are influenced by a range of factors. These include individual characteristics and behaviour, the physical environment, and the social and economic conditions. Some of these factors can be influenced by an individual's actions, such as lifestyle. Others, such as genetic make-up, cannot be changed. The social and economic circumstances that impact upon health and well-being – the conditions in which we are born, grow up, live, work, and age – are termed the 'social determinants of health' (CSDH, 2008). These factors have been described as 'the causes of the causes' of illness. For example, while smoking causes illnesses such as coronary heart disease and lung cancer, whether an individual is likely to start to smoke and then to successfully stop smoking is heavily influenced by social, economic, and environmental factors. It is important to take these social determinants into consideration when assessing health needs to ensure interventions are designed to address the causes of a health problem, rather than just its consequences.

The concept of need is often explained using four main categories identified by Bradshaw (1972). They are:

- *Normative need*: need based on expert opinion and determined by defined criteria, for example benefit levels.
- *Comparative need*: need defined by comparison with others who are not in need. For example, social deprivation in one area compared with that in another area that may be more or less deprived.
- *Felt need*: what people themselves say they need.
- *Expressed need*: need that can be inferred via people's demand for health services.

Health needs assessments are used to identify and analyse the health needs of a defined population. Cavanagh and Chadwick (2005) define health needs assessment as 'a systematic process of identifying priority health issues, targeting the populations with most need and taking action in the most cost effective and efficient way'. Health needs assessments are often undertaken by government agencies to better plan health services at the national and regional levels. Community organizations also undertake health needs assessments at the local or neighbourhood level to advocate for new services. Health needs assessments may be undertaken for a specific geographical area, such as everyone living in a defined neighbourhood, or for specific population groups, such as women with young children.

If a health needs assessment has been undertaken for the target population of your intervention, it is important to use this to design your proposed intervention from the outset. Important questions to clarify include:

- What does the health needs assessment tell you about the problem the proposed intervention seeks to address?
- How significant is this problem compared with other problems?
- What does the health needs assessment tell you about the proposed beneficiaries?
- What are their views about the problem the proposed intervention seeks to address?
- What does the health needs assessment tell you about inequalities in health?
- Will your proposed intervention address these inequalities or could it contribute to them?

Depending on the answers to these questions, you may need to adjust the focus of your proposed intervention.

It may be that a health needs assessment has already been undertaken for your target populations, but if there is no health needs assessment already available, you will need to undertake one. Guidelines on undertaking a needs assessment suggest that the following key stages be taken (WHO, 2001; Cavanagh and Chadwick, 2005):

Preparing for the health needs assessment

This involves deciding what the main population to be addressed will be; for example, all people living in a disadvantaged neighbourhood and any sub-population groups, such as children under five and their families living in a disadvantaged neighbourhood. It also requires bringing together the people who need to be involved, known as the stakeholders. This will include representatives of the population to be addressed, experts who know about the area and the target population, policy-makers and managers of local health and other service providers. Realistic aims and objectives for the health needs assessment then need to be established and the resources needed to carry it out identified.

Profiling

Profiling is the process of collecting and analysing information about the demographic make-up, health, and health needs of the population you are assessing. This information is likely to be made up of data from routine sources. This usually includes census data; data on births and deaths; health and lifestyle data and other data relating to the social determinants of health. Where sufficient data from routine sources are not available, you will need to collect new data. You will also need to collect information on what the population covered by the health needs assessment perceive to be their needs. Ways of collecting information and data include surveys (questionnaires and/or interviews), focus groups (small group discussions), and key informant interviews (interviews with individuals with special inside knowledge about the population).

Questions that need to be addressed during profiling include:

- How many people are in the target population?
- Where are they located?
- What data are currently available about them?
- What are the main common experiences and differences within the group?
- What are the health conditions and determinant factors affecting the health functioning of the population covered?

Prioritizing

The prioritizing stage of health needs assessment involves using the information you have gathered about the target population and comparing this with information about the current provision of services. This will enable you to identify health needs that are currently not being met and to select which interventions are most likely to have the greatest impact to improve health and well-being. Important questions to consider at this stage include:

- What services and interventions are currently being provided and what is known about the effectiveness of these approaches?
- What does the population whose health is being assessed prioritize as their most important health needs?

- What are the national and local priorities for health?
- What is the available evidence on interventions with potential for greatest health gains? (Using existing research to generate evidence about effectiveness is discussed later in this chapter.)

Identifying and engaging stakeholders

Individuals and agencies that have an interest in an intervention are often called stakeholders. Stakeholders can be divided into three types (Green and Tones, 2010):

- *Primary stakeholders*: potential beneficiaries of the intervention;
- *Secondary stakeholders*: those who may be involved in the intervention's delivery;
- *Key stakeholders*: those people without whom the intervention cannot go ahead.

Ethically, it is essential that you engage with people who may be affected by the intervention at an early stage in development. Potential beneficiaries should ideally be involved in both designing *and* implementing an intervention that aspires to meet their needs.

After identifying agencies, groups, and individuals who are potential stakeholders, the next step is to consider what they can potentially contribute to the intervention and how they can be actively engaged. The way you do this will depend on who they are and the nature of their interest in the intervention. Forms of stakeholder involvement include planning workshops, user-participation events, and partnership forums. Stakeholders require accessible information and facilitation for their participation to be meaningful. This should include information on the health needs assessment on which the intervention is based. Engagement with stakeholders takes time and needs to continue throughout the duration of the intervention. Engaging stakeholders in project completion is discussed further in Chapter 3.

 Activity 2.2

Imagine you are involved in designing a programme of interventions to reduce childhood obesity in your country. Think about who the stakeholders might be and divide these into primary, secondary, and key stakeholders.

Feedback

You should have identified children and their families in the target area as primary stakeholders. Secondary stakeholders could include schools, sports centres, youth centres, family doctors, food suppliers, funders of the intervention, and other organizations currently working with these beneficiaries. Key stakeholders should include the organizations without which the project could not go ahead, for example schools for a school-based intervention. You might have also included parents and carers because, without their support, it is questionable if some interventions could proceed.

Defining aims

Aims are broad statements about what change an intervention seeks to achieve. One way to define the aims of an intervention is to answer the following question: 'In what way do you want the target group to be different after the intervention?' As Chapter 1 discussed, overall health promotion aims are usually broad and achievable only through several complementary interventions being grouped together into a programme, rather than by one intervention alone. Each intervention needs to have clearly defined aims that contribute to those of the programme. For example, the overall aim of a healthy eating programme might be to bring about reductions in childhood obesity. The aim for a project making up one element of this programme, such as a school-based nutrition education project, might be to improve young people's knowledge about healthy eating. A project may have more than one aim.

Defining objectives

When you have decided on your intervention aim(s), you can define your objectives. Objectives describe how you will achieve your aim(s). A simple way of thinking about clear objectives is the SMART model. This stands for:

- **S**pecific: with clear, defined outputs;
- **M**easurable: you will be able to know when you have achieved these outputs;
- **A**greed: the outputs are agreed in advance;
- **R**ealistic: the outputs are not dependent on other factors that are unlikely to happen;
- **T**ime-limited: the outputs will happen within a set time.

Objectives should contribute directly to the achievement of the aim(s). A common error in developing objectives is to lose sight of the aims. The link between the aims and the objectives is subject to your theory of change, which will be explained later in the chapter. To ensure the objectives will contribute to the achievement of the aims, you will need to use your research on the evidence of how previous interventions have worked in similar settings and with similar groups.

Selecting intervention methods

After you have defined the needs the intervention seeks to meet and its aims and objectives for achieving this, you will need to decide which intervention method is most appropriate. Section 2 of this book discusses the methods used in health promotion interventions in more detail. When you go on to undertake your evidence review, you might highlight how effective different methods have been in achieving your proposed aims in other interventions. Depending on the need(s) your intervention is addressing, you may need to use more than one method. Interventions that use several methods to achieve change at different levels are discussed in Chapter 13.

When deciding on a method, you need to be clear about what theory supports the assumption that this method will achieve your aim(s). Theory can be defined as systematically organized knowledge applicable in a relatively wide variety of circumstances devised to analyse, predict or otherwise explain the nature or behaviour of a specified set of phenomena that could be used as the basis for action (Van Ryn and Heany, 1992). Because many of the theories used in health promotion have not been rigorously tested compared with, for example, theories used in the physical sciences, they are sometimes referred to as 'models'.

A detailed discussion of the different theories and models that are used to guide health promotion interventions is outside the scope of this book; however, Table 2.1 provides an

Table 2.1 Areas of change and the theories or models underpinning them

Areas of change	Theories or models
Theories that explain health behaviour and health behaviour change by focusing on the individual	• Health belief model • Theory of reasoned action • Transtheoretical (stages of change) model • Social learning theory

Theories that explain change in communities and community action for health	• Community mobilization
	  – Social planning
	  – Social action
	  – Community development
	• Diffusion of innovation

Theories that guide the use of communication strategies for change to promote health	• Communication for behaviour change • Social marketing
Models that explain changes in organizations and the creation of health-supportive organizational practices	• Theories of organizational change • Models of inter-sectoral action
Models that explain the development and implementation of healthy public policy	• Framework for healthy public policy – health in all policies • Health impact assessment

Source: Nutbeam *et al.* (2010)

overview of these. More explanation is provided in *Health Promotion Theory* which is part of the *Understanding Public Health Series* (Cragg *et al.*, 2013).

Theory can be used in the development of health promotion interventions in several ways. First, theory can be used to help understand a problem. It explains health-related behaviours and how these result from and interact with social, economic, and environmental conditions. It also helps to understand organizational dynamics and professional actions. In this way, a theory is used like a map to explain the nature of the issue you want to address, to consider how this relates to the populations you are working with, and to help you establish the broader context and other major factors influencing change. This is **what** the intervention will address and **who** it is addressing.

Second, theory can be used to help design an intervention. Theory makes explicit the role of health promoters and explores the thinking and beliefs that guide assumptions of how interventions can make an impact. A theory articulates what activities have to take place in order for an expected change to happen. It helps us to identify preconditions influencing pathways to change. This is **how** the intervention will achieve change and **when**.

Third, theory can be used to design the evaluation of the intervention. After articulating what the intervention seeks to change, for whom, how and when, you will be able to use this information to develop interim and final outcome measures. A theory can thus become a useful tool in demonstrating success and lessons learned.

Evidence review

There has been growing emphasis in recent years on the need to ensure that health interventions are evidence based – that interventions are made 'on the basis of the best available scientific data, rather than on customary practices or the personal beliefs of the health care provider' (Des Jarlais *et al.*, 2004: 361). This shift towards evidence-based practice began in the field of medicine in the early 1990s and has now been applied to public health, health promotion, and many other fields.

In planning a health promotion intervention, it is important to examine the evidence for the proposed intervention. In doing so, three key areas need to be explored. The first is around the intervention's *effectiveness*. This can be defined as whether it works to help produce favourable outcomes. In looking for answers about effectiveness, you will therefore need to identify studies that evaluate outcomes, both positive and negative, after exposure to an intervention similar to the one you are proposing. The second area is around the intervention's *feasibility* in your own setting. You will want to explore what is known about the circumstances or processes that help an intervention to work or impede effectiveness in a setting similar to that in which your proposed intervention will take place. The third area to explore is around an intervention's *acceptability*. When reviewing evidence of acceptability, emphasis is often placed upon the views or experiences of people likely to be at the receiving end of interventions, including target groups and the community in which the intervention will take place.

Using empirical research to inform health promotion planning is not straightforward. Research does not in general neatly divide interventions into those deemed 'effective' and those deemed 'ineffective'. There are a variety of reasons for this. Relevant evaluation research might not exist and what research there is may be of varying quality. This raises questions about the nature of evidence, such as what counts as 'evidence' and what is the 'best' evidence? This in turn raises questions about the research that underpins that evidence, such as how is the research funded and how it is interpreted and by whom?

In evidence-based medicine, there is often considered to be a hierarchy of evidence. This suggests systematic reviews and meta-analyses are the strongest form of evidence of effectiveness. Systematic reviews and meta-analyses are reviews of research that use an explicit approach to searching, selecting, and combining the relevant studies. In hierarchies of evidence, case reports are considered the weakest type of evidence. However, the concept of hierarchy of evidence is often problematic when appraising the evidence for social or public health interventions, as opposed to medical interventions. A matrix-based approach, which emphasizes the need to match research questions to specific types of research, may prove more helpful (Petticrew and Roberts, 2003).

In addition, given the huge quantity and breadth of research literature available, health promotion practitioners will rarely have the time to find and assess all of this and may find it difficult to know where to start. An information specialist or librarian should be able to provide guidance as to which bibliographic databases might be best suited for your needs, and can help with drawing up search terms and searching on databases. They can also help you identify other potential sources to search, such as health promotion journals and unpublished literature. Several international initiatives are now underway that focus upon the production and dissemination of high-quality reviews of research of relevance to health promotion. These include the Cochrane Public Health Group (http://ph.cochrane.org/).

Having identified potentially relevant evidence, it must be critically appraised to determine if it is valid and useful for planning your intervention. Given that there may not be consensus about the validity of evidence, it is important to have explicit criteria that can provide a consistent way of looking for indicators of quality across research studies. These criteria will depend on the type of evidence concerned, such as systematic review, outcome evaluation or process evaluation. Oliver and Peersman (2001) propose a range of questions that should be considered when reviewing evidence to help decide if and how it can be used to inform a proposed intervention (see Box 2.1).

Box 2.1 Questions to consider when reviewing evidence

For systematic reviews:
Are the results of the review valid?
Did the review address a clearly focused issue?
Did the authors select the right sort of studies for the review?
Do you think the important, relevant studies were included?
Did the review's authors do enough to assess the quality of the included studies?
Were the results similar from study to study?

What are the results?
What is the overall result of the review?
How precise are the results?

Will the results help locally?
Can the results be applied to the specific local population you are addressing?
Were all the important outcomes considered?
Are the benefits worth the harms and costs?

For outcome evaluations:
Are the results of the outcome evaluation valid?
Did the evaluation address a clearly focused issue?
Were the people receiving the intervention compared with an equivalent control or comparison group?
Were all the people who entered the evaluation properly accounted for and attributed at its conclusion?
Was the intervention described clearly?
Is it clear how the control group and experimental groups did or did not change after the intervention?

What are the results?
How large was the impact of the intervention?
How precise are the results?

Will the results help me?
Can the results be applied to the local population?
Were all the important outcomes considered?
Are the benefits worth the harms and costs?

For process evaluations:
Are the results of the process evaluation reliable? Does the study:
Focus on a health promotion intervention?
Have clearly stated aims?
Describe the key processes involved in delivering this intervention?
Tell you enough about planning and consultation?
Tell you enough about the collaborative effort required for the intervention?
Tell you enough about the materials used in the intervention?
Tell you enough about how the target population was identified and recruited?
Tell you enough about education and training?

What are the results?
Were all the processes described and adequately monitored?

Was the intervention acceptable?

Will the results help locally?
How can the results be applied to the local population?
Were all the important processes considered?
If you wanted to know if this intervention promotes health, what outcomes would you want to measure?

Source: Oliver and Peersman (2001)

Being able to identify and review evidence is an important skill for health promotion planners. However, it is also important to understand that having research evidence on the effectiveness, feasibility or acceptability of an intervention is only one piece of the picture. Local needs, available funding, and organizational characteristics will also influence whether an intervention is likely to be accepted and successful in promoting health.

 Activity 2.3

Imagine that you are developing an intervention to reduce smoking in your own country. Suggest the aim(s) and the objectives you would propose for the intervention.

Feedback

You should have reflected on what you have learnt about the difference between an aim and an objective. Your aim should be a broad statement that describes how the target group will be different after the intervention. An example of an aim for an intervention targeted at young people is 'reduced uptake of smoking in people aged 12 to 16'.

Your objectives should contribute to your aim(s) and be SMART (see the explanation of SMART in the section on defining objectives). Your objectives also need to relate to the method you have selected for your intervention.

The following are examples of objectives of an intervention targeting young people by working in schools:

- Increase knowledge among the target group about the immediate, as well as the long-term undesirable physiological, cosmetic, and social consequences of tobacco use through the provision of information via written materials and an interactive website (to be rolled out in ten schools over 2 years, reaching 15,000 young people).
- Provide training for 25 teachers involved in teaching the personal, social, and health curriculum in ten schools over 2 years on the reasons teens begin to smoke, such as a desire for maturity and acceptance, and how to offer them more positive means to achieve these same goals.
- Support the development of personal skills, such as assertiveness, confidence, and problem-solving skills, that will aid students in avoiding tobacco use as well as other risky behaviours through workshops as part of the personal, social, and health curriculum for the target group in ten schools over 2 years.

> • Develop a team of 30 peer educators to work in ten schools over 2 years to change the social norms about smoking, decrease social acceptability, and help students understand that most of their peers do not smoke.

Defining outcomes and outputs

After you have defined the intervention aims and objectives, you need to describe the outcomes and the outputs that will be generated. Outcomes are the changes that occur as a result of the intervention when the objectives are reached. Outputs are products, services, activities or attributes resulting from steps in the process of implementing the intervention. For example, an output of a vaccination campaign would be the number of people vaccinated, whereas the outcome would be the lower prevalence of the illness as a result of the vaccinations.

Defining outcomes and outputs is important, as they enable you to monitor the progress of the intervention to determine whether it is being implemented according to plan and to ascertain if it is having the intended impact on the target group. This will help you to identify any problems in implementing the intervention early on and to take action to rectify these. Defining outcomes and outputs is also crucial for evaluating the intervention. This is discussed in more detail in Chapter 4.

Identifying the required resources

Planning the intervention requires identifying the resources needed to implement it and thinking about where these will come from. They will include money and other resources such as staff and buildings. You will need to develop a budget for the intervention. A budget is a document that shows how much money you need in order to be able to carry out the activities required to meet your objectives. It allows you to identify the funding required and shows how you are proposing to spend it. As the intervention is implemented, the budget also enables you to see how much you have actually spent compared with how much you planned to spend and to make any necessary adjustments.

A budget breaks down planned expenditure into different categories of expenses often called budget headings or 'account codes'. Examples of budget headings include 'salaries', 'office costs', 'training costs', 'consultancy fees', and 'transport'. A budget also breaks down planned expenditure into time periods and gives the total cost. Most budgets divide planned expenditure into financial years. However, some budgets may be further broken down into quarters or months. Each agency or funder will have its own way of showing budgets. Budgets are discussed in more detail in Chapter 3.

Identifying risks and assumptions

Every project involves making assumptions and taking risks. The important thing is to understand what these are at the stage of planning the intervention so as to be able to manage them. Assumptions are factors outside the control of the project that will impact on the project if they are not realized. If an assumption is not met, other action will need to be taken. This action should be identified in advance. For example, an intervention to reduce obesity by improving healthy eating may have the availability of healthy food locally as an assumption. If it is not available locally, it will need to be brought in from elsewhere, which may affect the cost of the project.

A risk is the probability of something negative happening. If a risk is allowed to manifest, the success of the project will be threatened. Therefore, action needs to be taken to minimize risks and this should be built into the project plan. Potential risks include lack of or withdrawal of funding, insufficient support from key stakeholders, and failure to recruit to a crucial project post. Action to minimize these risks could include early and ongoing involvement of key stakeholders, including funders, and working with partner organizations to secure secondments for crucial posts. If a risk is identified that is likely to be realized because no action can be taken to minimize it, the project should be redesigned.

✎ Activity 2.4

Imagine you are designing an intervention to reduce unwanted pregnancy among teenage girls by using peer education in schools. What might the assumptions and risks be? What action might you take to minimize the risks?

Feedback

Examples of assumptions are that appropriate peer educators can be identified and are willing to speak in schools, and that family planning services are available for young women. An example of a risk is that head teachers will not be prepared to allow their schools to participate in the intervention. This risk could be minimized by early consultation with head teachers and their inclusion in the steering group for the intervention.

Planning for monitoring and evaluation

It is important to be clear about how you will assess whether the intervention or programme achieves its aims and objectives before you start implementation. This will enable you to put in place mechanisms for reviewing progress as it proceeds and evaluating it on completion, such as data collection and monitoring. Evaluation is discussed in detail in Chapter 4.

Planning for the intervention completion or scale-up

How an intervention is completed depends on its aims. Interventions with the aim of meeting ongoing needs may be handed over to another organization for continuation or scale-up. Alternatively, if the intervention is made up of finite, specified activities, it will be completed when these activities have been carried out. It is important to be clear about what the end point of an intervention is at the planning stage so the necessary activities to ensure successful completion can be defined and implemented. For example, an interim evaluation may be required before a project can be scaled up or additional funding may need to be identified.

Developing a project plan

The process of carrying out the different stages of planning of the intervention will generate information that needs to be presented in a structured and coherent way as an intervention plan. Before you proceed with the implementation of the intervention, you need to get approval for this plan. The type of approval you need will depend on where the funding for the intervention is coming from, the type of organization that is the lead agency, and whether the intervention has a project management or steering group. It is also important to give stakeholders involved in developing the intervention plan an opportunity to feed back on it, even if their approval is not formally required. Stakeholders are much more likely to actively support an intervention if they feel ownership of it.

Important factors in planning effective interventions

The following issues are important to consider when planning a health promotion intervention:

- As already outlined, it is essential to identify and involve stakeholders at an early stage. It may be a good idea to set up a working group to bring these together to work on planning the intervention.
- The intended beneficiaries, often described as the primary stakeholders, need to be involved in defining their own needs and interventions that seek to meet their needs. This important aspect of stakeholder engagement is often neglected.
- It should be made clear from the outset who is responsible for leading the process of planning the intervention. Given that several people will be involved in different ways, it is also important to be clear about who has responsibility for each stage of the planning process.
- The planning process needs to be proportional to the size of the proposed intervention. An intervention involving significant investment with a large target population will require more detailed planning over a longer period than a small-scale intervention.
- It is essential that the planning process is articulated in a written plan. The people involved are likely to change over the lifetime of the intervention, so it cannot be assumed those who implement the intervention will know about decisions that were taken at the planning stage.

Summary

This chapter has explained why health promotion interventions need to be properly planned if they are to be effective. It has introduced several models that have been developed to help conceptualize and carry out this planning. The process of planning a health promotion intervention involves a number of interrelated practical tasks that need to be articulated in a written plan. This planning is critical to ensuring the successful implementation and evaluation of the intervention. Chapter 3 discusses implementation in more detail, while evaluation is discussed in Chapter 4.

References

Bradshaw, J. (1972) A taxonomy of social need, *New Society*, March, pp. 640–3.
Cavanagh, S. and Chadwick, K. (2005) *Health Needs Assessment: A Practical Guide*. London: National Institute of Health and Clinical Excellence.

Commission on Social Determinants of Health (CSDH) (2008) *Closing the Gap in a Generation: Health Equity through Action on the Social Determinants of Health.* Final Report of the Commission on Social Determinants of Health. Geneva: World Health Organization.

Cragg, L., Davies, M. and Macdowall, W. (2013) *Health Promotion Theory.* Maidenhead: Open University Press.

Des Jarlais, D.C., Lyles, C. and Crepaz, N. and the TREND Group (2004) Improving the reporting quality of nonrandomized evaluations of behavioral and public health interventions: the TREND statement, *American Journal of Public Health*, 94 (3): 361–6.

Green, J. and Tones, K. (2010) *Health Promotion: Planning and Strategies.* London: Sage.

Green, L.W. and Kreuter, M.W. (2005) *Health Program Planning: An Educational and Ecological Approach.* New York: McGraw-Hill.

Maycock, B., Howat, P. and Slevin, T. (2001) A decision making model for public health advocacy, *International Journal of Health Promotion and Education*, 8: 59–64.

National Public Health Partnership (NPHP) (2000) *The Planning Framework for Public Health Practice.* Melbourne, VIC: NPHP.

Nutbeam, D., Harris, E. and Wise, M. (2010) *Theory in a Nutshell: A Practical Guide to Health Promotion Theories.* Sydney, NSW: McGraw-Hill.

Oliver, S. and Peersman, G. (2001) Critical appraisal of research evidence: finding useful and reliable answers, in S. Oliver and G. Peersman (eds.) *Using Research for Effective Health Promotion.* Buckingham: Open University Press.

Petticrew, M. and Roberts, T. (2003) Evidence, hierarchies, and typologies: horses for courses, *Journal of Epidemiology and Community Health*, 57: 527–9.

Van Ryn, M. and Heany, C.A. (1992) What's the use of theory?, *Health Education Quarterly*, 19 (3): 315–30.

World Health Organization (WHO) (1948) Preamble to the Constitution of the World Health Organization as adopted by the International Health Conference, New York, 19–22 June, 1946; signed on 22 July 1946 by the representatives of 61 States (Official Records of the World Health Organization, no. 2, p. 100) and entered into force on 7 April 1948.

World Health Organization (WHO) (2001) *Community Health Needs Assessment: An Introductory Guide for the Family Health Nurse in Europe.* Copenhagen: WHO Regional Office for Europe [http://www.euro.who.int/__data/assets/pdf_file/0018/102249/E73494.pdf?ua=1].

Further reading

Macintyre, S. and Petticrew, P. (2000) Good intentions and received wisdom are not enough, *Journal of Epidemiology and Community Health*, 54: 802–3.

Waters, E., Hall, B., Armstrong, R., Doyle, J., Pettman, T. and de Silva-Sanigorski, A. (2011) Cochrane update. Essential components of public health evidence reviews: capturing intervention complexity, implementation, economics and equity, *Journal of Public Health*, 33 (3): 462–5.

More information on ASTORs can be found on the Making it Count website [http://makingitcount.org.uk/planning; accessed 4 September 2014].

Implementing health promotion interventions 3

Will Nutland and Liza Cragg

Overview

Successful delivery of health promotion requires sound project management from planning through implementation to completion. Chapter 2 explored the different tasks involved in planning health promotion interventions. This chapter describes how to implement and complete interventions using key project management tools. In doing so, it also explains the importance of proper budgeting and budget monitoring and how to go about this. In addition, the chapter introduces tools that can help in keeping projects to schedule and in reporting progress to stakeholders. This chapter is designed and written as a 'how to' chapter on health promotion implementation and, as such, is not referenced in the same way as other chapters within the book. However, further relevant recommended reading is listed at the end of the chapter.

Learning objectives

After reading this chapter, you will be able to:

- describe the key tasks involved in effective implementation and management of health promotion interventions
- use different project management tools to facilitate the implementation and completion of health promotion interventions
- understand project management structures that assist in implementing interventions and programmes
- construct a chronogram and devise progress reporting systems
- prepare a project budget and monitor this

Key terms

Plan: A document that establishes the intended scope, aims, objectives, method, and activities.

Project management: The application of processes, methods, knowledge, skills, and experience to achieve the intervention or project objectives.

Strategy: An overarching plan informed by evidence, values, and theories that sets aims and describes how these will be achieved.

Implementing health promotion interventions using project management

Chapter 2 explained in detail how to plan health promotion interventions. It might seem that investing time and resources in planning the implementation of health promotion interventions is a luxury. However, establishing and describing in a written plan the aims, objectives, tasks, schedules, risks (and how to mitigate those risks), and having clear structures that clarify the roles and responsibilities for each stakeholder can save time and resources in the long term. In addition, having a plan for the intervention is crucial for its effective implementation and completion.

The implementation of health promotion interventions involves the utilization of project management tools. A project management approach tends to be most closely associated with industry and large companies or organizations. In those instances, complex project management processes are developed. Project management, however, does not have to be complex. There are different project management techniques and tools that are fit-for-purpose for different types and sizes of health promotion interventions. Although larger projects, particularly those being planned and implemented by governments or international agencies, might use project planning methodologies such as PRINCE2 (an acronym for **PR**ojects **IN** **C**ontrolled **E**nvironments), the tools described in this chapter do not require access to and training in such complex methodologies, and can easily be developed using basic computer systems (or even using pens, large sheets of paper, and sticky notes!).

This chapter now explains the key steps involved in effectively implementing and completing an intervention plan.

Setting up a project management structure

Establishing a clear intervention management structure is an essential element of project management. Conflicts and confusion can be mitigated by having clear structures, with defined roles and responsibilities. This is especially important if an intervention or programme involves multi-agency collaboration. Although structures will differ by organizations and programmes, a common structure is one that has project boards, a management or steering group, a project manager, and a project team.

Project boards

Increasingly, projects are delivered by partnerships made up of organizations from different sectors. Organizations and sectors have different ways of working and individuals have priorities and commitments to their own organizations. Therefore, it is important to build commitment to, and a shared understanding of, the project among those involved. One way of doing this is to develop a project board made up of the key individuals from the stakeholder organizations. Some planning processes also identify a *project sponsor* – someone senior who has overall responsibility and accountability for the project, and who supports the project manager.

Management or steering group

Complex or large projects may also require a project management or steering group. These will usually include the senior managers of the organizations involved in the project and can also include other stakeholders, such as beneficiaries. The role of a project management or steering group is to oversee and review the project's progress, provide accountability, and ensure senior commitment. Generally, the group meets regularly throughout a project's implementation. It might approve the project plan and budget and any subsequent amendments. Although establishing such a group may seem like introducing an unnecessary layer of bureaucracy, it can be a useful way of avoiding conflict where there are complex interactions of agencies.

In many cases, a project comes from an idea at a multi-agency meeting. It may be discussed in several forums and different organizations may sponsor research into needs, a feasibility study, and participation events. But before project implementation can commence, a decision should be taken as to who is the lead agency. This does not imply the lead agency must find all the required resources or take all the responsibility. However, to ensure good coordination, one agency must take responsibility for project management.

It is good practice to establish terms of reference for management or steering groups so that all stakeholders are clear about their roles and how the group will operate.

Project manager

When the lead agency has been established, an individual from that agency is usually assigned the role of project manager. The role of the project manager is crucial to the success of a project. This person coordinates the project, collates and disseminates information on progress, and coordinates the project team. The work involved in being the project manager is commensurate with the size and complexity of the project, but it is essential that the project manager has sufficient time and resources to carry out the role. For this reason, the function and responsibility should be included in that individual's formal work plan.

Project team

Developing a project team also requires capacity-building. Capacity-building is action to ensure the necessary resources, expertise, and commitment exist for the project's successful implementation. It may include training for members of the project team and staff in partner organizations on the skills needed to implement the part of the project in which they are involved. It could also involve team-building for the project management or steering group to build understanding of and commitment to the project. Capacity-building is also essential for the sustainability of the project.

If you need additional skills or capacity to implement the project, you may need to recruit new employees. When recruiting new employees, it is important to be clear about what the overall role of the new staff member(s) will be and how this relates to the project's aims, what specific tasks they will be required to undertake, and how they will be managed and supported. This should be laid out in a job description. You also need to develop a person specification that describes the skills, qualifications, and experience the new staff member(s) will need to have to carry out the job successfully. To get the right person for the job, it is essential you develop a job description and person specification before you begin recruitment. Recruitment should be undertaken in such a way that all potential candidates are given equal opportunities.

Developing an organogram

An organogram, or organizational chart, is a visual diagram that shows the structure of an organization, or a number of organizations within a shared programme of work, and the relationship and responsibility between different positions and roles. An organogram might also include a brief description of each position or role and the task each will perform. Developing an organogram for a health promotion intervention or programme will assist in clarifying the roles of staff, volunteers, stakeholders, steering groups, and project groups and, where appropriate, to whom each of these are accountable. These diagrams can be simple and follow a traditional hierarchical structure. More commonly, organograms, especially if a programme involves multiple stakeholders, will be more complex, with lines of responsibility running between different stakeholders. Figure 3.1 provides an example of an organogram from a multi-agency project proposal to reduce tuberculosis (TB) in a prison setting. Table 3.1 describes the responsibilities of the key staff members in the project.

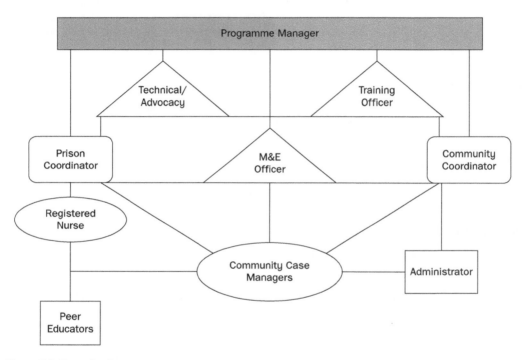

Figure 3.1 Example of an organogram.

✎ **Activity 3.1**

For a project with which you are familiar or which you have read about, try to create an organogram, linking in the key staff, volunteers, and other key players.

Feedback

You might have found that there were multiple links between different staff and stakeholders and it is common for there to be multiple relationships between key players. When this is the case, it is essential to know where responsibilities start and finish, and where decisions are made.

Table 3.1 Examples of key responsibilities of staff

Position	Responsibilities
Programme manager	Oversee programme implementation, manage staff, liaise with stakeholders
Administrator	Provide administrative support to programme staff
Prison coordinator	Oversee prison programme, training, and supervision
Registered nurse	Training and assistance in the implementation of prison TB screening, diagnosis, and treatment
Community coordinator	Oversee community integration programme, training, and supervision
Monitoring and evaluation officer	Collection of baseline data, establish monitoring systems, compile reports and liaise with evaluators
Training officer	Establish programme training system
Technical/advocacy	Provide expertise and advocate for structural reform
Community case managers	Provide support to released prisoners with TB
Peer educators	Provide education on TB/HIV and support peers within prison

Defining and timetabling activities

Chapter 2 explained the importance of defining aims and objectives for your intervention as part of the planning process. Implementing the intervention requires defining the activities that will achieve the objectives and a timescale for these activities. In doing so, remember that some activities will be dependent on the completion of others. It is important to be clear about the interdependence of project activities at this stage because, if one activity is delayed, it may result in the delay of other activities.

Critical path method/analysis

Undertaking a critical path analysis (CPA) is one way of establishing the interdependence of activities, and is a tool commonly used by project managers as a means of establishing the shortest possible time to complete a project. A CPA works by establishing four essential sets of information:

1 All of the activities necessary to complete the project;
2 The time required (or duration) to complete that activity;
3 The dependencies between each activity (that is, if one needs to be completed before another can commence); and
4 End-points for activities such as milestones or deliverables.

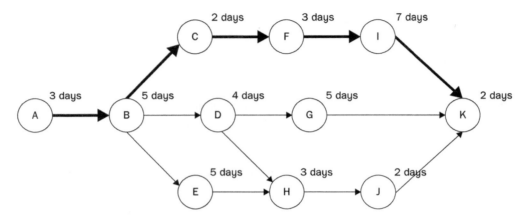

Figure 3.2 Example of a critical path.

By mapping this information, the analysis can calculate the longest path to complete the project and its activity, and the earliest and latest each activity can commence or be completed without the project taking any longer. This also establishes the activities that are *critical* and are on the longest path and the activities that have *float* and can be delayed without making the total project duration any longer. The combination of activities that take the longest time to complete are known as the *critical path*. This is the shortest time in which the overall project can be completed. Thus, any delay on any of the activities on that critical path will delay the project as a whole. Knowing the critical path assists a project manager in knowing where to target resources if a project faces delays. Projects can have a number of parallel critical paths that may combine at points in the project.

Figure 3.2 provides an example of a critical path for a project. Each circle represents a stage in the completion of an activity. The numbers beside each circle represent the estimated number of days to complete each task. The critical path is the path along the top of the diagram (the thicker arrows). Even if other steps are completed sooner, the whole task cannot be completed in under 22 days.

Milestones and chronograms

When you have defined the activities and the order in which they need to be delivered, you need to set 'milestones' for the project. Milestones signal the completion, or progress points, of key activities that indicate progress in the project. They enable you to see easily if the project is, or isn't, on track. A chronogram is a clear way of presenting the project activities and milestones. These are also sometimes referred to as 'Gantt' charts. Figure 3.3 outlines a chronogram for an intervention that lasts three years with activities down the side.

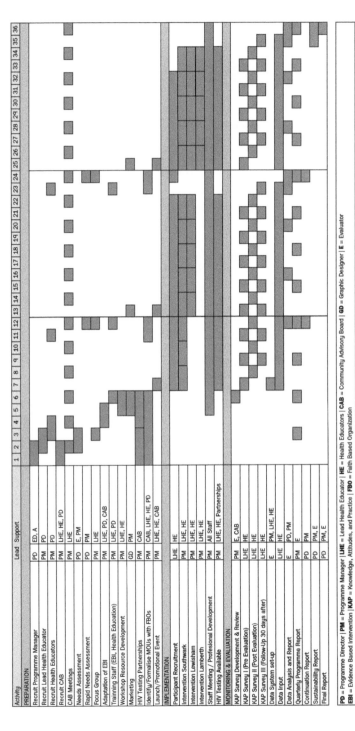

Figure 3.3 Example of a chronogram for a 3 year intervention.

PD = Programme Director | **PM** = Programme Manager | **LHE** = Lead Health Educator | **HE** = Health Educators | **CAB** = Community Advisory Board | **GD** = Graphic Designer | **E** = Evaluator
EBI = Evidence Based Intervention | **KAP** = Knowledge, Attitudes, and Practice | **FBO** = Faith Based Organization

Activity 3.2

Read the case study below. Then map out the key milestones in the case study and use these to develop a chronogram for the programme of interventions.

Case study

You are a manager of an organization that aims to increase the levels of physical exercise in the local population and you are applying for funding to undertake a mass media intervention and outreach programme for your local population.

The mass media intervention must run for six months and it must undergo formative evaluation (pre-testing) prior to its launch. A mass media intervention of this size costs £180,000 in media placement and the formative evaluation takes one month to complete and costs £10,000.

The developers of the mass media intervention (an external contracted company) will need two months of initial development time before it goes to formative evaluation. They will then need one further month of re-development time between sending their work for pre-testing and receiving feedback from the evaluation team. The development team's total cost for work on the project is £45,000 – this does not include the research costs.

The outreach programme must accompany the media campaign and cannot start before the media campaign. Your funders want to see a minimum of 120 units of outreach. Each outreach unit has to be undertaken by two outreach workers and they cost £100 each per session. The workers will need to be trained on their first day and the training package, which takes a month to develop, will need to be prepared before they start work. The training development package will cost £5000. You should allocate a further £5000 per month for pedometers and materials to be distributed during outreach sessions.

In addition, the funders want to see an outcome evaluation of the whole project. You know that the evaluation of projects of this size takes six months and will cost £30,000. The evaluation work will commence in the last three months of the media intervention. Funders also require a sustainability report. This will take two months to complete and cannot commence until the evaluation report is submitted. The sustainability report will be developed by you along with a consultant. The consultant charges £8000 per month.

You will take overall management of the project – this will take 20% of your time each year on a total salary of £48,000 per year. You will also need to recruit a project worker on a salary of £36,000 per year. You should add salary on-costs for you and the project worker of 10% of your salary. Your organization will also charge organizational on-costs of £45,000 to cover administrative and organizational costs. Recruitment for the project worker should commence from the point of confirmation of the funding and recruitment will take 3 months. The recruitment costs will be £5000 and the worker is needed until the completion of the programme. None of the work on any part of the programme can begin until the project worker is in post. The project worker must organize and hold a stakeholder meeting in the month they come in to post and should hold one at the start of the media campaign, one at the end, and a final one when the sustainability report is launched at the end of the programme. You should also allocate a contingency budget of £15,000 to cover any unforeseen expenditure.

Feedback

Your chronogram should look similar to Figure 3.4. You will see that some of the activities are overlapping and take place concurrently and some are dependent on others being completed. Note that the outreach training development is only dependent on recruitment of the project worker, so could commence prior to month 7. A more detailed chronogram might include some of the assumed activity undertaken by the project worker such as ordering outreach materials, organization of outreach events or activity, and booking of media activity.

Activity	**Month number**																	
	1	2	3	4	5	6	7	8	9	10	11	12	13	14	15	16	17	18
Recruit worker	X	X	X															
Design activity				X	X		X											
Pre-testing						X												
Training development							X											
Media campaign								X	X	X	X	X	X					
Outreach activity								X	X	X	X	X	X					
Outcome evaluation											X	X	X	X	X	X		
Sustainability Report																	X	X
Stakeholder engagement				X				X					X					X

Figure 3.4 Example of a simple chronogram for Activity 3.2.

Early wins

When setting a timetable for project activities, consider if it is important to include some 'early wins'. Early wins are visible successes at the start of a project that will build commitment to the project on the part of stakeholders. However, early wins should not take focus away from the longer-term progress of the project, and you should be aware of the risks of promising to commissioners or stakeholders early wins that cannot then be achieved.

Assigning responsibilities

Specific responsibilities for the project activities need to be assigned to the relevant members of the project team; these should ideally be integrated into their work plans to ensure they happen. When developing a work plan, it is also important to consider whether any professional development may be required in order for the staff member to meet the objectives and to include the method and timescale for meeting these development needs in the work plan.

Evaluation

When planning the project activities, it is essential you include the evaluation of the project. You need to decide what evaluation questions you will seek to answer, what methods you will use, and what information you will need. You cannot leave it until the project has started to decide what type of evaluation you will do, as by then it may be too late to collect the necessary information. If external evaluators are being used, they should be included at the earliest stages of project planning: their insight will be essential. Chapter 4 discusses intervention evaluation in more detail.

Meeting quality standards

As part of defining the project activities, you need to think about how you will ensure the quality of the project activities and outcomes. There may be internal or external quality standards that are applicable to the project. For example, many agencies have minimum user standards or charters. There may also be legal requirements regarding informed consent or confidentiality. Many professions have professional standards that will need to be applied to the intervention activities (for example, medical or nursing standards; therapeutic or counselling ethical standards) or quality standards that apply to the delivery of certain types of services (for example, clinical services).

Consideration needs to be made in the planning for the health and safety of staff and volunteers working on the programme. Additional training may be required, or buildings brought up to standards to meet legal safety codes. Provision may need to be made to ensure that workplaces meet equality and access legislation, for example by ensuring that people with physical impairments are able to access workplaces.

Preparing and monitoring the budget

A budget is a document that shows how much money you need to carry out the activities required to meet your objectives. It allows you to identify the funding required and how you are proposing to spend it. By monitoring the budget you are also able to see how much you have actually spent compared with how much you planned to spend and make any necessary adjustments.

Different categories of expenditure called budget headings or 'account codes' can be created that break down planned expenditure into things such as 'salaries', 'office costs', 'training costs', 'consultancy fees', and 'transport'. Activities are costed separately in a budget and the cost is put in the relevant budget heading or account code. Each agency or funder will have its own account codes. These indicate how the agency breaks down its expenditure in its annual accounts. Generally speaking, the bigger an agency's expenditure, the more detailed its account codes will be.

A budget also breaks down planned expenditure into time periods and gives the total cost. Most budgets divide planned expenditure into financial years. However, some budgets may be further broken down into quarters or months.

Figure 3.5 provides an example of a simple budget and Figure 3.6 shows a more detailed one. A budget needs to contain enough detail for it to be useful in managing the project but not so much detail that it is unwieldy. The level of detail should be commensurate with the size of funding involved, with larger sums of money requiring more detailed breakdown. It is normally drafted by the project coordinator using information provided by members of the project team on the components of the project they will implement. Most large organizations have a finance manager who will provide support, test assumptions, and critically appraise the draft budget. The project management or steering group, or the relevant finance manager or director for the lead implementing agency, is usually required to approve a draft budget before it becomes final.

Once a detailed budget has been drafted, it is essential to review the proposed intervention outputs of the project. It is not uncommon for outputs to be adjusted if initial assumptions about the costs of delivering the outputs were unrealistic. If alterations have to be made, these should also be discussed by the steering group and, where appropriate, negotiated with the funder of the work, if funding has already been secured.

Costs	Projected Expenditure		
	Year 1	Year 2	Year 3
Total staff costs	**55000**	**56100**	**57222**
Project manager x 1	25000	25500	26010
Secretary x 0.5	10000	10200	10404
Trainer x 1	20000	20400	20808
Total office costs	**7150**	**3938**	**4477**
Office supplies	500	600	800
Office equipment and hardware	4000	500	500
Office rent	1500	1530	1561
Office maintenance and insurance	400	408	416
Communication costs and posted fees	750	900	1200
Total peer educator costs	**15400**	**12400**	**12400**
Recruitment costs	3000	0	0
Consultant to train and support 12 days @ £200 a day	2400	2400	2400
Expenses for peer educators 50 @ £10 a day for 20 days	10000	10000	10000
Total training costs	**7500**	**7500**	**5500**
Training session materials	2500	2500	500
Training room costs 20 days @ £100 a day	2000	2000	2000
Refreshments for training session 20 days @ £50 a day	1000	1000	1000
Creche for training session 20 days @ £100 a day	2000	2000	2000
TOTAL COSTS	**85050**	**79938**	**79599**

Figure 3.5 Example of a simple budget.

STAFF / CONSULTANT

Salaries	Year	Year 1 %	Monthly	# Months	Staff	Total	Year 2 %	Salary (*)	Months	Staff	Total	Year 3 %	Salary (*)	Months	Staff	Total	Programme Total
STAFF																	
Programme Director	£ 42,000	25%	£ 3,500	12	1	£ 10,500	25%	£ 3,605	12	1	£ 10,815	25%	£ 3,713	12	1	£ 11,134	£ 32,454
Programme Manager	£ 34,000	100%	£ 2,833	10	1	£ 28,333	100%	£ 2,918	12	1	£ 35,020	100%	£ 3,006	12	1	£ 36,071	£ 99,424
Lead Health Educator	£ 29,000	25%	£ 2,417	8	1	£ 4,833	50%	£ 2,489	12	1	£ 14,935	50%	£ 2,564	12	1	£ 15,383	£ 35,151
Health Educator (seasonal)	£ 24,000	20%	£ 2,000	6	9	£ 21,600	20%	£ 2,060	12	19	£ 43,436	20%	£ 2,122	10	19	£ 80,628	£ 146,164
Total Salaries Full Time						£ 43,667					£ 60,770					£ 62,593	£ 167,030
Total Salaries						£ 65,267					£ 154,706					£ 143,222	£ 363,194
Payroll and Benefits (10%)						£ 4,367					£ 6,077					£ 6,254	£ 16,703
Total Personnel cost						£ 64,633					£ 160,783					£ 144,481	£ 379,897
Organizational On-Cost (20%)						£ 13,927					£ 32,157					£ 29,896	£ 75,479
Total Staff						£ 83,560					£ 192,940					£ 179,377	£ 455,877
CONSULTANT																	
Evaluator	£ 75,000	100%	£ 6,250.00	4	1	£ 25,000	100%	£ 6,438	4	1	£ 25,750.00	100%	£ 6,631	4	1	£ 26,522.50	£ 77,273
Graphic Designer	£ 30,000	20%	£ 2,500.00	2	1	£ 1,000	20%	£ 2,575	1	1	£ 515	10%	£ 2,652	1	1	£ 265.23	£ 1,780
Total Consultants						£ 26,000					£ 26,265					£ 26,788	£ 79,053
Total						£ 109,560					£ 219,205					£ 206,165	£ 534,929

OPERATIONAL COST

OPERATIONAL COST	Unit Cost	# Units/mo	# Months	Total	Unit Cost	# Units/mo	# Months	Total	Unit Cost	# Units/mo	# Months	Total	TOTAL
Office Expenses	£ 80		12	£ 960	£ 80	2	12	£ 1,920	£ 80	2	12	£ 1,920	£ 4,800
Computer Equipment	£ 300	5		£ 1,500	£ 300	5		£ 1,500	£ 300	5		£ 1,500	£ 4,500
Workshop materials	£ 80	6	1	£ 480	£ 80	2	12	£ 1,920	£ 80	2	10	£ 1,600	£ 4,000
Promotional Event	£ 500	1	1	£ 500	£ 500	2	1	£ 1,000	£ 500	2	1	£ 1,000	£ 2,500
Community Advisory Board	£ 200	6	1	£ 1,200	£ 200	6	2	£ 2,400	£ 200	6	2	£ 2,400	£ 6,000
Focus Group	£ 300	1	1	£ 300	£ 300	1	1	£ 300	£ 300	1	1	£ 300	£ 900
Food	£ 75	20	6	£ 9,000	£ 75	40	12	£ 36,000	£ 75	40	10	£ 30,000	£ 75,000
Transportation	£ 9	40	6	£ 2,160	£ 9	80	12	£ 8,640	£ 9	80	10	£ 7,200	£ 18,000
Training	£ 45	10	6	£ 2,700	£ 45	10	12	£ 5,400	£ 45	10	12	£ 5,400	£ 13,500
Rent	£ 60	20	6	£ 7,200	£ 60	40	12	£ 28,800	£ 60	40	10	£ 24,000	£ 60,000
General Liability Insurance	£ 40	4	12	£ 1,920	£ 40	4	12	£ 1,920	£ 40	4	12	£ 1,920	£ 5,760
Staff Recruitment	£ 5,000	1	1	£ 5,000	£ 2,000	1	1	£ 2,000	£ 2,000	1	1	£ 2,000	£ 9,000
Total				£ 32,920				£ 91,800				£ 79,240	£ 203,960
Contingency Reserve (5%)				£ 1,646				£ 4,590				£ 3,962	£ 10,198
TOTAL Operational Cost				£ 34,566				£ 96,390				£ 83,202	£ 214,158
TOTAL Programme				£ 144,126				£ 315,595				£ 289,367	£ 749,087

(*) Inflation rate = 3%

Figure 3.6 Example of a detailed budget.

The process for developing a budget varies from agency to agency. Generally, the key steps are as follows:

- Describe the activities required to achieve the project's objectives;
- Obtain information on the costs of each activity (some funders will put an upper limit on what these costs can be);
- Cost the activities and present these costs in the categories given as budget headings or account codes;
- Prepare a budget narrative that describes what the figures are based on;
- Ask finance colleagues to check the draft budget;
- Get approval for the draft budget.

Providing a narrative is very important. Imagine you come to take over the role of project manager in the middle of a project. How will you know where the figures come from? You should include:

- a breakdown of global figures;
- assumptions about beneficiary numbers and consumption;
- assumptions about risks;
- the basis on which you have estimated costs, for example: '4 newsletters at £5000 each'; 'two part-time peer educators at £10,000' each.

The following points are useful tips to help you prepare a budget:

- Familiarize yourself with the budget requirements of the funder and lead implementing agency before you start;
- Include provision for inflation and other predictable cost increases where a project continues over several years;
- Ensure that you have included any overhead costs for your organization, such as office costs, insurance or a contribution to the cost of human resource services, administrative support or IT systems – and ensure that these costs are in line with the contribution limits of your funders;
- Include the full costs of employing staff and not just their salary – employers might have to pay health insurance or social security contributions;
- Begin as early as possible so you have enough time to involve the project team;
- Try to get consensus – it is very difficult to manage a budget if some of the people involved say they never agreed the costs in the budget;
- Label different drafts of the budget clearly and if you circulate them to colleagues, keep track of the master copy;
- Do not change costs without consulting the person who gave them to you or you may find you misunderstood what the costs were based on and are left with insufficient funding in the budget;
- Ask for technical advice – you cannot know what everything costs.

Once you have developed the budget, you need to secure the necessary funding. Funding may be available from within the overall budget of the lead implementing agency or from a national government programme of which the project forms part. Alternatively, it may be necessary to raise money for the project from grant-giving bodies, commissioning agencies, trusts or partner organizations. Increasingly, health promotion projects tend to be funded by a variety of different sources with a single project often receiving funds from government, partner organizations, and trusts.

✏ **Activity 3.3**

Return to the case study given in Activity 3.2. First, try to create budget headings for the key areas of expenditure and identify the total that will be spent in the programme for each budget heading. Then, using the budget examples above to guide you, construct a more detailed budget for the programme, breaking expenditure down by quarters (3 month blocks). You might want to refer back to the chronogram you constructed to identify when expenditure might occur.

Feedback

Your budget should be similar to Figure 3.7, with budget headings that capture the key areas of proposed expenditure. Note that the project worker is not working for the

Budget heading	Total expenditure
Project manager (20% of £48k annual salary for 18 months)	£14,400
Project worker (Annual salary of £36,000 for 15 months)	£45,000
10% on costs on salaries	£5,940
Project worker recruitment costs	£5,000
Sessional outreach staff	£24,000
Outreach materials	£30,000
Sessional training package	£5,000
Development of mass media intervention	£45,000
Pre-testing	£10,000
Media placement	£180,000
Outcome evaluation	£30,000
Sustainability report	£16,000
Contingency	£15,000
Organizational on-costs	£45,000
TOTAL	**£470,340**

Figure 3.7 Example of a budget for Activity 3.3.

whole duration of the project (the first 3 months are taken up by recruitment), so ensure that their salary is adjusted accordingly.

Figure 3.8 provides an example of what you might have created for the more detailed budget. You should note that the total budget for each quarter is different. This is because activity, and expenditure related to that activity, is not divided equally across each quarter, with a concentration of activity and expenditure in quarters 3 and 4 when most of the outreach and media activity occurs.

	Q1	Q2	Q3	Q4	Q5	Q6	TOTAL
Project manager	2400	2400	2400	2400	2400	2400	14400
Project worker		9000	9000	9000	9000	9000	45000
10% on costs	240	1140	1140	1140	1140	1140	5940
Recruitment	5000						5000
Outreach staff			8000	12000	4000		24000
Outreach materials			10000	15000	5000		30000
Training			5000				5000
Media development		30000	15000				45000
Pre-testing		10000					10000
Media spend			60000	90000	30000		180000
Outcome evaluation				10000	15000	5000	30000
Sustainability report						16000	16000
Contingency	2500	2500	2500	2500	2500	2500	15000
Organizational on-costs	7500	7500	7500	7500	7500	7500	45000
TOTAL	17640	62540	120540	149540	76540	43540	470340

Figure 3.8 Example of a more detailed budget for Activity 3.3.

Monitoring and reporting progress

Monitoring progress against the original plans is an essential component of project management. Project monitoring information will be required to check the progress of the project and to ensure compliance with applicable quality standards. Monitoring should focus on assessing whether the key activities are occurring. Data from monitoring may also be used in the overall evaluation of the project. You must be clear about how monitoring information will be collected, who will collect it, and who will review it before the implementation of the project proceeds. This is discussed in further detail in Chapter 4.

Most project boards and management or steering groups will be expected to review ongoing monitoring data and to be made aware of issues or concerns with delivery of milestones. A simple tool for visualizing milestone progress is the RAG (Red, Amber, Green) status criteria, shown in Table 3.2. This simply identifies if a project board or management group needs to take action on progress of a milestone's achievement by coding each milestone with a colour in a progress report.

A project highlight report is another key reporting tool that allows top-level progress on a project or programme to be reported to the project board. A highlight report should provide clear and accurate information on a project's status, together with recommendations for progressing through risks and issues that provides an audit trail for the project. A highlight report should contain the key elements as summarized in Table 3.3.

Completing the project

An essential element of project management is having an agreed process for project completion – also known as an exit strategy. It may be that the nature of the project means that it will come to a definite end at a particular point – for example, if it is to undertake a piece of research. Alternatively, the project may involve the establishment of a service that will need to be sustained. You need to identify actions you must take to ensure the sustainability of the project at this stage. These could include seeking funding, handing over the project to a different agency or building in income generation.

Evaluating whether the project achieved its objectives

You need to assess to what extent the project has achieved its aims and objectives it set itself and answer the evaluation questions set. This is discussed in more detail in Chapter 4.

Table 3.2 RAG status

Colour	Status
BLACK	Milestone has been achieved
RED	Not on track – severe impact on project's delivery and requires urgent escalation
AMBER	Not on track but under control
GREEN	On track and under control

Table 3.3 Key elements of a project highlight report

Element	Definition
Period covered by the report	
Overall status of the project	Assessed against the RAG status criteria – based on assessment of progress against the project plan, milestones, and resources used
Key risks	These risks will be updated based on those identified in the project plan
Key issues	Any new or major issues that the board needs to be appraised of
Key milestones achieved in last period	Landmark points of completion indicating progress on project
Non-completion in last period	Milestones that have not been completed together with proposed actions to address shortfalls
Forecast for next period	An identification of milestones due for the next period and views on their achievability
Financial status	A summary of the actual spend against planned spend and actions to be taken to resolve discrepancies

Managing staff exits

Line managers of staff working on the project need to undertake regular performance review meetings with staff throughout its course. Formal feedback on performance needs to be provided to staff in the form of a staff appraisal annually and at the completion of the project. Staff members should be given the opportunity to say how they think they performed as part of the appraisal. The project manager may be taking on a new role after the completion of the project. It is essential they undertake staff appraisals before they move on.

Handing the project over or finishing the project

You should have identified any necessary action to ensure the project's sustainability when you planned the project's activities. Depending on the nature of the project, it may be handed over to another organization for continuation. Handing it over will involve inducting the new staff, explaining the management of premises, and taking steps to ensure continuity of service.

Alternatively, if the project was by nature of a fixed term or if it has achieved its objectives, its purpose may have been achieved and it is now finished. Finishing a project will itself require some action depending on the nature of the project. For example, research may involve the production and presentation of a report of the research. Alternatively, finishing a project may necessitate the disposal of assets, terminating staff contracts, and making arrangements for other agencies to take over any residual functions.

Disseminating information

The final task of project management will usually be to disseminate information about the project to ensure knowledge transfer about the project's learning. A final report may be required by a project funder or the lead implementing agency. Even if a final report is not formally required, it may be useful to produce one in order to ensure that the learning gained in the course of the project is not lost when the manager and others involved move on to different roles.

Stakeholders will have given time, resources, and commitment to the project and it is important to consider how they will be informed about the project's success or learning. This might be done through websites, forums, meetings or publications. It is also important to consider sustainable and long-term knowledge transfer methods that take the learning from the project and make it available to future interventions. This might take the form of policy guidelines, training events or resources, workshops or learning tools.

Critical factors for success in implementing health promotion interventions

Implementing and completing health promotion interventions can be a complex task. Multi-agency working, competing priorities of agencies, and working to tight budgets and timelines, along with unforeseen factors, can make the task more complex still. Planning well, and planning well in advance, is an essential element of success. Further critical factors for success include that the intervention:

- has a clear plan, with aims and objectives that are achievable, feasible, and realistic;
- is adequately resourced and has the relevant human resources to deliver the interventions;
- has a transparent and appropriate project management process, with clearly defined expectations and responsibilities, especially with regard to multi-agency programmes;
- engages with relevant stakeholders throughout the planning, implementation, and completion of the intervention;
- has identified potential risks to the intervention and strategies to mitigate those risks.

Summary

This chapter has described the importance of following a project management approach in the implementation and completion of health promotion interventions and programmes. Key project management tools assist in planning activities and milestones, and in reporting the progress of activity. Other tools assist in mapping the key players involved in planning and delivering projects, and their respective responsibilities. Project management is crucial to ensure that projects are implemented as planned, to time and to budget.

Further reading

Executive Agency for Health and Consumers (EAHC) (2011) *Project Management in Public Health in Europe* [http://ec.europa.eu/chafea/documents/health/leaflet/project_management2.pdf].

Green, J. and Tones, K. (2010) *Health Promotion: Planning and Strategies*. London: Sage.

More information on planning and implementing health promotion can be found on the Making it Count website [http://makingitcount.org.uk/planning; accessed 9 November 2014] and the Knowledge, Will and Power website [http://kpw.org.uk/planning; accessed 9 November 2014].

4 Monitoring and evaluating health promotion interventions and programmes

Will Nutland and Meg Wiggins

Overview

Evaluation and monitoring are important components of planning, implementing, and completing a health promotion intervention. This chapter discusses outcome and process evaluation, and the importance of formative evaluation in the development of interventions. It describes how to establish outcomes and outputs, together with tools to assist in designing evaluations and monitoring progress. The chapter outlines three key evaluation methods and how to apply them to the evaluation of different types of interventions. Finally, the chapter explores some of the practical issues in undertaking evaluation and monitoring, and the appropriate role of health promotion providers and planners in evaluation.

Learning objectives

After reading this chapter, you will be able to:

- explain the purposes of evaluation and monitoring and the role they play in health promotion planning
- understand outcome evaluation and process evaluation and how they interact
- establish intervention outcomes and outputs and set indicators for them
- select evaluation designs and methods that are appropriate for the health promotion intervention concerned
- understand who should undertake intervention evaluation and the role of a health promotion planner or provider in evaluation and monitoring

Key terms

Evaluation: The critical assessment of the value of an activity.

Formative evaluation: An evaluation that takes place before the launch of an intervention, or during its implementation, with the goal of improving its implementation or functioning.

Outcome evaluation: An evaluation that seeks to establish whether or not an intervention brought about its strategic aim.

> **Process evaluation**: A method of gathering and analysing information that helps to establish how and why an intervention brought about change.
>
> **Monitoring**: The systematic collection and collation of information about the performance of an intervention or programme as it progresses. Monitoring must be based on targets set and activities agreed during the planning phases for an intervention.

Why is evaluation important?

The evaluation of health promotion activity helps to establish if an intervention, or programme of interventions, has met its stated aims, and how those aims have or have not been met. In a climate where public health activity is increasingly evidence based and evidence driven, knowing how to use and understand evaluation and monitoring is an essential part of health promotion planning.

Being able to understand evaluation and monitoring methods is important for health promotion planners because:

- Funders and commissioners of health promotion usually insist that interventions include an element of evaluation to demonstrate that their funding has been well spent;
- Evaluation and monitoring assist in refining and developing interventions, and are an integral part of a health promotion planning cycle;
- Evaluation of health promotion activity adds to existing bodies of evidence that inform the development of new interventions, hones existing interventions, and enables replication of interventions and transferability to appropriate settings or target groups.

Chapter 1 explained some of the important concepts involved in developing health promotion interventions. It stressed that an intervention needs to be sufficiently described for it to be evaluated. Intervention descriptions should include the key qualities of an intervention: what is done (objectives and methods), where it took place (the setting), with what (resources), to achieve what change (aims), and for whom (target), as well as the behavioural choice the intervention seeks to influence. Chapter 2 provided practical guidance on how to develop a plan for a health promotion intervention that includes all these qualities, and Chapter 3 explored how to implement and manage such an intervention. Identifying these qualities is essential to enable evaluation because they specify the key qualities of the intervention that can be evaluated. These qualities are: feasibility, costs, acceptability, coverage and access, relevance, effectiveness, and efficiency. These are described in more detail in Box 4.1.

Box 4.1 Qualities of interventions to determine through evaluation

Feasibility: Is it possible to undertake the intended objective in the specified setting with the finite resources? (Can it be done?)

Cost: What resources are needed, including human resources, equipment, and money? What is the overall cost per target group member who encounters the intervention?

Acceptability: What does the target group think of the objectives, particularly in the setting? What do other stakeholders think of the intervention?

Coverage and access: How many, or what proportion, of the target group encounter the objectives? How do they differ from the target group members who do not encounter them? What are the biases in access to the intervention?

Relevance: Do the target group require the change that the intervention aims to achieve? Has this change already been achieved by the target group before they encounter the objectives? Do the specific needs the intervention is seeking to address correspond to those of the target group?

Effectiveness: Do the objectives bring about a change for the target group? Which target group members who encounter the intervention benefit the most and which the least?

Efficiency: Were all resources used in the intervention necessary to bring about the change that occurred? How does the intervention compare to others that bring about the same amount of change for the same amount of people?

Source: CHAPS Partnership (2011)

Types of evaluation

In order to explore these seven qualities, evaluations need to be appropriately designed. In this chapter, we explore three types of evaluation – outcome, process, and formative evaluation – which are described below. These types of evaluation can be used to explore any or all the seven qualities of an intervention described above.

Outcome evaluation

Outcome evaluation seeks to tell us whether or not an intervention has brought about its strategic aim, such as a benefit or change within a population. Health promotion activity can aim to reduce or prevent diseases, illness or other biological outcomes, some of which, such as obesity, are associated with disease, while others, such as teenage pregnancy, are regarded as negative because of the impact on the health and social well-being of the parents and the child. Some interventions will aim to promote health in a positive sense, such as increasing physical activity or improving mental health. Measuring whether or not negative outcomes have been averted or positive outcomes have been achieved will be important for those planning and commissioning health promotion interventions. As such, it is important to identify whether health promotion interventions are effective (Bonell *et al.*, 2003).

Process evaluation

Process evaluation seeks to establish how an intervention has or has not brought about its aim, and whether it may have brought about other outcomes (unintended outcomes). Process evaluation can assist in determining why an intervention was or was not effective, how the intervention was undertaken in reality, and how the intervention might be undertaken in another setting or context. Process evaluation can provide:

- A clear description of the intervention being delivered (rather than the one that was planned);
- An indication of the feasibility, fidelity, and quality of the intervention;
- How acceptable the intervention is to the target group and other stakeholders, including those delivering the intervention;
- The actions that caused these changes brought about by the intervention;
- Contextual influences that impacted on the delivery of the intervention;
- The replicability of the intervention (could the intervention be transferred to other settings or target groups).

Process evaluations should describe how interventions are planned and implemented in sufficient detail for others to judge whether and how they might replicate the intervention. It is not uncommon for published evaluations to provide rigorous evidence on effectiveness but less robust information on the intervention itself and how it was undertaken (Ellis *et al.*, 2003).

Although it is common for process evaluation to be used at a formative stage of intervention planning (see below), it is important not to disregard the utility of process evaluation throughout a cycle of delivering an intervention. Ongoing process evaluation can be used to continuously refine and improve an intervention as it is being implemented (Stewart, 2000), and can aid understanding of how and why the outcomes were achieved (or not as the case may be).

Outcome versus process evaluation

Outcome and process evaluations are not rivals. Although it is common for process evaluation to be used at an early 'formative' stage of an intervention to refine that intervention, and to then focus on outcome evaluation at a 'summative' stage, they can be used together, as is seen in the case study below. Process evaluation might also be used to inform the transfer or scale-up of an intervention. Case study 4.1 outlines how a process evaluation was used to better understand the outcome findings.

Case study 4.1: Using process evaluation to understand the outcomes of a UK diabetes intervention

The CASCADE study was a randomized control trial (RCT) of a psycho-educational intervention for young people with diabetes in the UK. It explored whether attending a series of facilitated education groups with other young people with diabetes (and their parents) would help to improve the control young people had over their blood sugar levels.

The study had an extensive multi-method process evaluation that ran for the 4 years of the RCT. The aims of the process evaluation were to: (1) describe the provision of the CASCADE intervention and assess the feasibility of providing this within a standard diabetes clinic setting for a diverse range of young people; and (2) to build on and help explain trial outcome findings and to provide information on how the intervention might be modified. The process evaluation used a range of both qualitative and quantitative methods, including: observations of education sessions; interviews with a subsample of young people, parents, and clinic staff; questionnaires to assess perceptions of the intervention; attendance data; and case note review.

The RCT found that the education groups were not effective in improving the young people's control over their blood glucose levels. The process evaluation was key in determining why this was the case. The critical factor was that the intervention proved administratively difficult for the clinic teams to organize, so a large proportion of recruited young people were not offered education groups or reminded to attend. Families found it difficult to attend the group sessions that were offered because of school and work commitments. Only 53% of the young people attended any of the group sessions. Those with the most difficulty controlling their blood sugar levels were least likely to attend group sessions. Those who did attend the education group sessions found them helpful and credited them with helping control their diabetes. The process evaluation findings suggest that the concept of the group education sessions was one that should be explored further, but the organizational and administrative arrangements would need to be altered to make the groups better attended.

Note: The study was funded by the NIHR-HTA and carried out by a multi-institutional team (University College London Hospital, London Institute of Education, London School of Hygiene and Tropical Medicine, and the School of Pharmacy) (Christie *et al.*, 2013).

Formative evaluation

Formative evaluation usually takes place prior to the launch of an intervention (or programme) or during the implementation phase, and includes any action that assists in shaping and forming the intervention. Formative evaluation might include literature reviews and other forms of evidence appraisal, needs assessment, and pre-testing of intervention ideas and expectations with the intended target audience. In addition, formative evaluation can:

- Assist in developing an intervention description by defining and describing what the intervention will look like;
- Establish the feasibility of the intervention and establish if the intervention will 'work' in the real world (for example, Is the intervention culturally appropriate? Would the target group be prepared to encounter the intervention in the proposed setting?);
- Identify if the proposed intervention is acceptable both to the target group and those delivering the intervention;
- Test the proposed logic model or theory of change by establishing if the intervention could lead to the target group doing what the intervention set out to get/enable them to do.

Case study 4.2: Formative evaluation to inform an antenatal intervention in East London

In one multi-cultural area of London with high deprivation rates, a health care provider identified that a large proportion of pregnant women were not accessing antenatal care until later than was desirable (after 13 weeks pregnancy). Late access to antenatal care is linked to greater health concerns for the mother and the baby.

To identify the reasons behind the problem and to determine the best intervention to address it, a formative research study was conducted. This involved a systematic review of literature on existing interventions targeting early uptake of antenatal care; analysis of health records to determine the profile of those late in accessing care; focus groups with women via community organizations and maternity staff; and interviews with pregnant women and new mothers.

The findings were presented to a workshop of key local stakeholders, maternity experts, and researchers. Those attending came to a consensus about what types of interventions might be most locally appropriate solutions to address the problem. Three interventions were funded and subsequently evaluated.

Note: A team from the University of East London, Institute of Education, and City University conducted the research (Harden *et al.*, 2011).

Monitoring health promotion interventions

Monitoring involves the ongoing collection of information about an intervention that assists in understanding the intervention's performance against a pre-determined plan. Data collected from monitoring is frequently used to establish and report on the progress of an intervention, and can be used to assist in determining whether the intervention has met its aims. All health promotion interventions should have a monitoring scheme as part of their overall plan. The monitoring scheme should determine the output indicators that the intervention is being measured against (see below). As part of the intervention planning, it is important to establish how monitoring data will be collected; how the data will be recorded (for example, by pen and paper, on a computer system); and how and when monitoring data will be reported (including who the data will be reported to and for what purpose). It is common for programmes to establish output or service delivery 'targets' (for example, 20 workshops to be delivered every month) and monitoring systems will help to establish if these 'targets' have been met.

It is important to be realistic about the quantity and type of monitoring data that is planned to be collected. Those providing health promotion interventions frequently collect monitoring data themselves, and it is important that the amount of data collected does not compromise the integrity of the intervention itself. With interventions that encounter very large numbers of people, it is common for 'snap shot' monitoring data to be captured at regular intervals, rather than trying to collect monitoring data from every encounter.

Monitoring data are often collated, analysed, and reported on a regular basis by those managing the intervention to see how the intervention is progressing. For example, monthly or quarterly progress reports are likely to include data on how many people have used the services provided by the intervention. However, it is important to stress that this type of routine monitoring is very different from an evaluation. An evaluation will certainly use the data collected through this routine monitoring, but it will be analysed by an external evaluator and supplemented by additional information.

Outcomes and outcome indicators

For an intervention to be evaluated, it is necessary to identify the outcomes of the intervention. Outcomes are directly related to the aim of an intervention and are the tangible result of having undertaken the intervention. An outcome might be an increase in knowledge in a given population; a decrease in a behaviour within a target group; or an increase in the number of people booking or accessing a health service. Outcomes are what changes in a particular population as a result of encountering an intervention. Outcomes might be different across sub-groups within a target population (for example, a desirable outcome of a teenage pregnancy programme might be increased knowledge on the part of all teenagers within an area, but for that increase to be more profound in girls who are under 16). Outcomes might also be expressed as incremental change over time (for example, an increase in knowledge in one class of a school in year 1 of the project, an increase in knowledge across a whole school in year 2, and by year 3 an increase in knowledge across a town).

Outcome indicators are a way of expressing how a change is measured. This might be the actual change, such as a percentage increase in knowledge, or the numbers of people who booked into a health service within a set period of time. As it is not always possible to identify an actual measure, such as when the outcome of the intervention will not be seen for years after the intervention, a proxy measure of change can be identified. A measure that correlates with or predicts change might also be used.

✐ Activity 4.1

Identify an example of an intervention when a proxy outcome indicator might be used. What might you use as a proxy outcome indicator?

Feedback

There is a broad range of examples of interventions when proxy outcome measures, rather than actual measures, will be used. Proxy measures are often used when it is impractical to measure actual outcomes because the outcomes will only be seen in years ahead. For example, interventions targeting young girls to reduce teenage pregnancy might be unable to measure pregnancy rates in those girls in years to come, so might use a proxy measure instead such as age at sexual debut as an outcome indicator. Interventions to reduce alcohol use might adopt hospital admissions for alcohol-related harms as a proxy measure.

Output and output indicators

For interventions to be monitored, outputs need to be identified. Outputs relate directly to the outcomes, and thus the strategic aim, and describe the tangible and meaningful activities that are undertaken to achieve the outcome. These outputs are sometimes described as 'deliverables'. Intervention outputs might include the interactions that take place (for example, group work, outreach sessions, help-line conversations), media materials (for example, leaflets, website pages, adverts) or any other type of health promotion activity (for example, policy document, training event).

Output indicators describe the level of activity that is undertaken. This might be the numbers of interactions that take place; the numbers of people who are accessing an intervention; the frequency of training events held and the numbers of people attending.

To summarize, outcomes relate to evaluation and outputs relate to monitoring.

✎ Activity 4.2

Going back to the example given in case study 4.2, identify the outcomes for the programme of interventions. What might some of the outcome indicators be? What might some of the outputs and output indicators be?

Feedback

Outcomes for the intervention in case study 4.2 include an increase in awareness of the need for early uptake of antenatal services, and an increase in uptake of antenatal services. An outcome measure might be the percentage of pregnant women booking into the service in the first 13 weeks of pregnancy. An output might be a community engagement event, and output indicators could include the number of events held, how many people attended, and the number of people in the specific target group who attended the event.

Developing an evaluation and monitoring framework

Chapters 2 and 3 discussed the importance of including a framework for capturing and recording evaluation and monitoring data as part of the process of planning and delivering a health promotion intervention. Having identified specific aims, objectives, outcomes, and outputs for an intervention, and then identifying the outcome and outputs indicators, it is important to identify the methods by which the information will be collected, and who will be responsible for collecting and collating that information. A range of different tools has been developed to capture this information, with one example of a template given in Figure 4.1. Figure 4.2 provides an example of a completed template for a programme to increase awareness of HIV and sexual health in Nairobi.

Intervention aim	Outcome	Indicator	Data source	Responsibility
Objective	Output			

Figure 4.1 Evaluation and monitoring framework template.

Source: adapted from Charities Evaluation Services (2013).

Aim (and outcomes)	Outcome indicator	Evaluation description
To increase the target group's awareness of HIV and sexual health	An increase in men reporting knowledge on how HIV is transmitted and prevented	Men asked to complete a short 5 question questionnaire prior to the intervention.
	An increase in men reporting that they know where and how to access an HIV test	Post intervention, men asked to complete another KAP survey. When men agree to provide contact details a follow-up KAP survey is emailed to them 3 months after the intervention
	An increase in men reporting they have had an HIV test and/ or a sexual health screening at one of the project's recommended clinics	
		Staff in the project's recommended clinics record referral data
To increase access to condoms and lubricant	An increase in men reporting that they have easy access to condoms and lubricant, or who report having condoms and lubricant with them	Survey collects data as does outreach worker's field notes on men refusing condoms because they already have access to them

Setting	Five bars in eastern Nairobi
Target group	Men who have sex with men under 45 who live, work or socialize in Nairobi

Objectives (and outputs)	Output indicator	Monitoring description
To undertake five outreach sessions each week of 4 hours at each of five bars	25 sessions per week	Records kept by outreach workers indicating dates and duration of sessions and venue.
To approach a minimum of 150 men each week and offer an outreach session	150 men approached	Session records indicate numbers of approaches, encounters, duration of encounters and numbers of materials distributed. Field notes kept by workers capture knowledge needs of men encountered.
To invite a minimum of 100 men each week to complete a pre-intervention survey	100 men approached	
To undertake an outreach session of a minimum of 5 minutes with a minimum of 100 men each week	100 men encountered	Basic demographic data is recorded by outreach workers to indicate if intervention is reaching the men in the target group.
To invite all men who encountered an outreach session and who completed a pre-intervention survey to complete a post-intervention survey	75 men approached 50 pre and post KAP forms completed	
To distribute 500 condom and lubricant packs each week	500 packs distributed	

Figure 4.2 Example of evaluation and monitoring framework to increase the awareness of HIV and sexual health in Nairobi.

Evaluation design

When considering evaluation design, it is important to consider the research questions you are attempting to answer and the resources available to you. Randomized control trials (RCTs) are usually considered the 'gold standard' in evaluating health care interventions. The key distinguishing feature of an RCT is that study participants are randomly allocated to receive one or other of the alternative treatments under study. However, there is debate as to how appropriate RCTs are in the evaluation of health promotion interventions when proper randomization may be hard to achieve and there are many compounding factors that can affect outcomes. In addition, RCTs are expensive and require large groups of participants, so it is likely that only evaluations of large interventions will have the resources and time to conduct such a trial. Most health promotion activity will have to draw on other designs.

A common problem in health promotion evaluation is the wish to carry out the most comprehensive evaluation possible, targeting a number of research questions and incorporating a sophisticated design with multiple methods. Although this may be entirely appropriate for some interventions, for others it can be a case of 'too much, too soon'. A complex and large-scale evaluation can be expensive to carry out and will require staff and infrastructure to do so effectively. It is important to weigh up the resources available and the questions you want to be answered.

Attempting to carry out an over-ambitious evaluation can, in some circumstances, result in that evaluation being aborted because there are not enough resources to complete it. It is far more sensible to be 'up front' from the outset with the funders of research, programme directors, and other decision-makers about the capacity for evaluation and the types of appropriate research questions that can be answered regarding the intervention. As discussed earlier, sometimes the priority is to do a relatively simple process evaluation well, rather than a complex outcome evaluation badly.

Using the appropriate evaluation methods or tools

Evaluation data can be collected in a variety of ways. The method depends on the type of evaluation design being used, practical considerations relating to the characteristics of the people involved, and the resources available to undertake the evaluation. The sensitivity of the information being requested might also determine the method used. Participants might be more willing to answer questions about sexual activity or drug use, for example, if the evaluation method offers a greater degree of confidentiality. These aspects will be discussed further under each method below. We will discuss in detail three of the most commonly used evaluation methods: surveys, interviews, and focus groups. These methods can be used separately or in combination. There are a number of other evaluation methods that can be used to gather data, including case studies, observations, and photographic or video diaries.

Surveys

Surveys involve asking (usually) relatively large numbers of participants a number of preset questions in a standard way. Surveys can be self-completed by participants using questionnaires (paper or digital) or participants can engage in structured interviews with evaluators (in person or over the telephone). Surveys can use 'closed' questions with a predefined set of answer options to provide quantitative data, and 'open' questions that allow the participant to give an answer in their own words, usually to provide qualitative data.

Surveys can be used to explore outcomes or processes. For instance, in the evaluation of a mass media smoking cessation intervention, a survey might examine outcomes by asking questions about knowledge of the effects of smoking on health, current smoking behaviours or health status. To examine process, the survey may explore people's awareness of or views on the intervention and how they encountered it. Surveys usually provide simple answers to questions – useful for quantifying an issue but not for providing in-depth information about motivations or aspirations and similar 'why' questions (e.g. exploring why people start to think about quitting or how the campaign influenced them).

Evaluators need to take into account the circumstances of their potential participants when planning a survey. Literacy problems or other factors may impede the use of self-completion questionnaires and therefore necessitate structured interviews. However, the latter will be more time-consuming. Even surveys relying on self-completion question-naires still require considerable time and staffing resources for the design, production, distribution, and collection of questionnaires, as well as data input and analysis. The recent development and increasing popularity of on-line survey tools has made undertak-ing surveys and analysing their results much less time-consuming. However, relying solely on these surveys could introduce bias into the results, as some members of the target group may not have access to the internet.

Semi-structured interviews

A key evaluation method for gathering in-depth information is interviewing, where an eval-uator engages in a 'conversation' with an interviewee that is less structured than the sorts of surveys discussed above. The interviewer asks questions but does not restrict the interviewee to answering according to preset options and allows the participant consider-able leeway in guiding the course of the exchange. The interviewer can probe or introduce new questions when it is felt that more information on a certain topic would be useful. This allows for the collection of qualitative data and a more in-depth exploration of the interviewee's experiences and perceptions. Interviews can be used to gather in-depth data about outcomes but are more often used to explore people's experiences and views on process. Data from semi-structured interviews are not used to quantify but rather to describe and explain.

Interviews are semi-structured when the interviewer uses a specific topic-guide to steer the discussion around set themes, using probes if necessary. Interviews are usually audio- or video-recorded and transcribed, or written notes are taken. Some interviews may be enhanced with the use of visual prompts or diagrams. It will sometimes be essential for interviews to be conducted by an individual with whom the interviewee can identify, such as someone of the same age, gender, sexual orientation or ethnic group. In other cases, it may be that differences in identity are acceptable or even potentially more useful to interviewees. Interview-based research is usually very time-consuming but does not involve such vast production or distribution costs as survey research.

Focus group discussions

Focus group discussions are another method for gathering in-depth, qualitative data from a relatively small number of participants. Rather than interviewing one person at a time, a group of approximately 6 to 12 people are brought together and asked questions, again in a semi-structured way. Rather than exploring individual views in depth as interviews do, focus groups allow a group of peers to share their views and allow the researchers to observe group interaction. This method can be used to examine social norms and ways that these can influence attitudes and behaviours (though it cannot measure behaviour itself). Combining focus group and interview data can enable evaluators to compare different points of view, different motivations, and the degree of consensus on a topic. Focus groups should not be regarded merely as a time-saving way to interview lots of people; the questions that can be answered by each method are different. Although running a focus group may not take much time, they are usually very time-consuming to organize beforehand and to transcribe and analyse afterwards. Although people sometimes feel more comfortable in discussing certain topics when talking among their peers rather than on their own in an interview, sometimes they do not. Evaluators should be aware of the following issues when considering the appropriateness of focus groups:

- cultural sensitivities about discussing certain issues in a group setting;
- power relations within groups whereby the views of some dominate those of others;
- confidentiality; and
- difficulties in setting up groups across widely dispersed populations.

Like interviews, focus groups are most commonly used to explore process but can also contribute substantially to formative evaluation by scoping or pre-testing interventions before their release. Focus groups can be audio- or video-recorded, or notes taken. It is helpful for two research team members to be present: one to facilitate the discussion and the other to observe and take notes about the interaction.

 Activity 4.3

You wish to carry out a process evaluation of a peer education intervention to promote exercise among men over 50. In this evaluation, you want to explore whether the intervention was delivered as planned, whom it reached, and how acceptable it was to the peer educators, their peers, and those planning and training the peer educators. What methods would be most appropriate to use?

Feedback

A variety of methods are available to you. You might consider using a combination of the following:

- Questionnaire completed by peer educators (how confident they felt in delivering peer education; how motivated they were; their perception of the intervention – what worked well, what was hard, and what would have helped);

- The survey could be supplemented with individual semi-structured interviews with the peer educators or focus group discussions with them;
- Interviews with trainers of peer educators and planners of the programme (how well they felt the training went; challenges to delivering it; perception of how peer educators received training and accepted new role);
- Focus groups with recipients of peer education to explore their experiences of receiving the intervention.

The importance of ethical issues

Informed consent

Participants should only be involved in an intervention *or* its evaluation (including what and how data will be collected and used) on the basis of their prior, informed consent. Where individuals are allocated randomly to the intervention or comparison group, this should also be done only after participants have given informed consent. The information provided should be clear and easy for potential participants to understand and they should be given the opportunity to ask questions. Issues of confidentiality should be explained. It should be made clear that participants' consent is voluntary and that they can choose to withdraw at any time during the evaluation. Even in situations where it is not practical for participation in the intervention to be voluntary (for example, participation in mass media campaigns delivered within a cluster RCT), participants should still be asked for their voluntary, informed consent to participate in data collection for the evaluation.

Storage and use of data

The storage of data that may contain sensitive and confidential information should be considered before data collection. Information that personally identifies individuals should be kept separate from their process and outcome data. For example, each participant can be assigned a code that is used to identify their questionnaires or interview transcripts, rather than their name. Any contact details provided by participants should be kept separately and all data should be stored securely. Finally, data must be reported both accurately and transparently. When reporting, data should be sufficiently anonymized so that individuals cannot be identified from their responses. Where this anonymity is not possible, the individuals should be given the opportunity to vet their responses to ensure they are happy for them to be made public. Most countries have legislation that describes how data should be collected and stored, and this must be complied with.

Ethical approval

Medical research involving human participants requires ethical approval. This means a proposal for the research needs to be considered by a formally constituted research ethics committee before it can begin. For the purposes of research governance, 'research' means the attempt to derive generalizable new knowledge by addressing clearly defined questions with systematic and rigorous methods. Whether an evaluation counts as research depends on its scope and purpose. However, it is always advisable to check with the relevant health care commissioner/provider or academic body whether ethical approval is required for an evaluation.

Who should undertake health promotion intervention evaluation?

There is not universal agreement on who should commission and conduct the evaluation of health promotion interventions. Everyone involved in the planning, design, and delivery of health promotion activities can make use of evaluation techniques and engage in evaluative activities to improve interventions. Health promotion practitioners should be well versed in evaluation techniques to assist in planning interventions, including being able to understand if an evaluation of another intervention is credible and to understand how they might use the findings of evaluations to inform their own intervention planning. In addition, health promotion planners should be able to distinguish between different evaluation methods and be able to apply relevant methods to their intervention planning.

It might be tempting, especially if funding is scarce or a health promotion intervention is small, for those delivering health promotion interventions to also undertake its evaluation.

✎ Activity 4.4

Consider the pitfalls of an intervention planner or provider also being responsible for the evaluation of that intervention. Make a short list of these potential problems.

Feedback

Those providing an intervention will not be independent and will have a vested interest in marketing the intervention. As such, even if the evaluation is undertaken well, it may lack credibility. Evaluation findings are often used to 'sell' or promote an intervention, or to justify its continued funding, and there may be a temptation to 'spin' the findings to make them appear more favourable. Intervention evaluations are resource intensive and may take time, energy, and focus away from intervention delivery. Interventions and evaluations are likely to have different aims and outcomes and this will present a challenge if the same individual or team undertakes them. It might also be that an intervention or planner does not have the appropriate skills to undertake evaluation.

So, best practice suggests that intervention delivery and intervention evaluation should be undertaken independently, and major funders of health promotion programmes will often commission intervention evaluation separately from intervention delivery to increase the independence of evaluation. This does not mean, however, that planners and providers of health promotion should not be involved in any evaluation activity.

Resourcing evaluation activity

Evaluation activity can have significant costs in terms of time, money, and energy. Commissioners of health promotion activity may insist upon evaluation and stipulate the evaluation activity that is expected and the percentage of the budget that should be allocated to evaluation. Whatever the level of activity that is decided upon, evaluation should be a central part of the health promotion planning process. It should not be an afterthought and needs to be appropriately resourced. Poorly funded evaluation can seriously limit the amount that can be learnt about a programme. Those who commission, develop or conduct programmes need to consider carefully the risks and benefits of a poorly resourced evaluation.

Disseminating evaluation findings

If and how evaluation findings are disseminated can, in part, be dictated by the funder or commissioner of a health promotion intervention. As has already been discussed, commissioners are often keen to publish findings of flagship interventions if the evaluation is favourable, but might be less keen for less favourable findings or 'lessons learnt' to be made public. As part of a health promotion planning process, it can be useful to establish at the start how evaluation will be disseminated, and how learning will be shared.

Evaluation findings can be published in peer-reviewed journals, either by health subject area (for example nutrition, sexual health, diabetes) or by health professional specialism (e.g. nursing, therapy, physical training). However, such journals are not always accessible to planners, may not be especially timely in the publication of their results, and are likely to focus on larger-scale interventions and evaluations.

Health promotion planners can consider a range of other methods that target and tailor their evaluation dissemination, including conferences, seminars, webinars and workshops; guidelines and policy formation; newsletters; and newspaper and magazine articles.

Consideration should be given to how stakeholders, especially end users of the intervention being evaluated, are informed of the evaluation findings. Increasingly, funding bodies will insist on strategies to engage and disseminate to end users any evaluation findings, and this should be seen as good practice, however small the evaluation or intervention.

Summary

Evaluation and monitoring of health promotion interventions and programmes are important components of health promotion planning. Evaluation is necessary to examine not only the outcomes but also the process of planning, delivery, and receipt of interventions. Outcome evaluations and process evaluations are two commonly used health promotion evaluation types – but they are not rivals and will often be used in tandem. Evaluations can collect data via methods such as surveys, interviews, and focus groups. Pitfalls to avoid when undertaking evaluations include being overambitious, trying to evaluate your own intervention, undertaking an evaluation too late, and neglecting ethical responsibilities.

References

Bonell, C.P., Bennett, R. and Oakley, A. (2003) Sexual health should be subject to experimental evaluation, in J. Stephenson, J. Imrie and C.P. Bonell (eds.) *Effective Sexual Interventions: Issues in Experimental Evaluation*. Oxford: Oxford University Press.

CHAPS Partnerships (2011) *Making it Count 4: A Collaborative Planning Framework to Minimize the Incidence of HIV during Sex between Men*, 4th edn. London: Sigma Research.

Charities Evaluation Services (2013) *About Monitoring and Evaluation*. London: Charities Evaluation Services.

Christie, D., Thompson, R., Sawtell, M., Allen, E., Cairns, J., Smith, F. *et al.* (2013) Structured, intensive education maximizing engagement, motivation and long-term change for children and young people with diabetes: a cluster randomised controlled trial with integral process and economic evaluation – the CASCADE study, *Health Technology Assessment*, 18 (20): 1–202.

Ellis, S., Barnett-Page, E., Morgan, A., Taylor, L., Walters, R. and Goodrich, J. (2003) *HIV Prevention: A Review of Reviews Assessing the Effectiveness of Interventions to Reduce the Risk of Sexual Transmission*. London: Health Development Agency.

Harden, A. *et al.* (2011) *Achieving Equity in Access to Antenatal Care: A Pilot and Development Study for a Research Programme to Understand and Overcome the Barriers*. Final report to NIHR. London: University of East London.

Stewart, W. (2000) Use of process evaluation during project implementation: experience from the CHAPS project for gay men, in M. Thorogood and Y. Coombes (eds.) *Evaluating Health Promotion Practice and Methods*. Oxford: Oxford University Press.

Further reading

Charities Evaluation Services (2013) *Tools and Resources*. London: Charities Evaluation Services.

Harden, A. and Gough, D. (2012) Quality and relevance appraisal, in D. Gough, S. Oliver and J. Thomas (eds.) *An Introduction to Systematic Reviews*. London: Sage.

Thorogood, M. and Coombes, Y. (eds.) (2000) *Evaluating Health Promotion Practice and Methods*. Oxford: Oxford University Press.

SECTION 2

Methods used in health promotion

Healthy public policy

Matt Egan

5

Overview

Research has repeatedly demonstrated the importance of socio-economic and environmental conditions in influencing the health of individuals and populations (Marmot *et al.*, 2010). Government policies are major drivers of social conditions, and of public health and health inequalities. This chapter describes how social policies beyond the health sector – such as those affecting housing, transport, income, trade, and welfare – can be incorporated into public health strategies by using Healthy Public Policy (HPP). The chapter discusses key concepts underpinning HPP, and explores some of the challenges involved in its delivery.

Learning objectives

After reading this chapter, you will be able to:

- explain how population health and health inequalities are created by social determinants outside the health sector
- describe how Healthy Public Policy (HPP) attempts to advance public health goals through joint action across a range of public policy areas
- describe some of the key challenges to delivering HPP and how these might be overcome

Key terms

Health inequalities: Differences in health experience, status, and outcomes between countries, regions, and socio-economic groups.

Public health: All organized measures to prevent disease, promote health, and prolong life among the population as a whole.

Social determinants of health: Conditions that affect people's health such as their working and living environments, income, social networks, and social position.

What is healthy public policy?

In 1986, the World Health Organization (WHO) issued the Ottawa Charter for Health Promotion. This Charter called on governments to:

Build Healthy Public Policy

Health promotion goes beyond health care. It puts health on the agenda of policy makers in all sectors and at all levels, directing them to be aware of the health consequences of their decisions and to accept their responsibilities for health. (WHO, 1986)

Healthy Public Policy (HPP) is a response to the widely held understanding that non-health sector policies and interventions have an important role in creating the conditions for health. Access to health services remains a vital contributory factor in explaining the health status and outcomes of populations but, viewed in the more holistic terms of HPP, it represents just one in a long list of determinants that affect people's living standards, opportunities, and quality of life throughout the life course (Marmot *et al.*, 2010). Public policy on these broader social determinants of health is formulated and implemented through 'non-health sector' political and administrative infrastructures with goals, cultures, and personnel that are distinct from those related to health service delivery. Public health practitioners must find ways of influencing these broader policy areas to ensure that health is on the agenda of all relevant policy-makers 'in all sectors and at all levels' (WHO, 1986). Chapter 6 of this book provides more information on how advocacy can be used to do this.

 Activity 5.1

What social determinants are likely to affect health? Are there particular government policies (outside of the health sector) you can think of in your own country that have the potential to improve health or to harm it for different social groups?

Feedback

The WHO Commission on Social Determinants of Health defined the social determinants of health as the conditions in which people are born, grow, live, work, and age. These circumstances are shaped by the distribution of money, power, and resources at global, national, and local levels (WHO, 2008). They include a wide range of factors:

- Availability of resources to meet daily needs
- Access to education
- Early years services
- Access to health care and other services
- Job training
- Employment opportunities
- Access to recreational and leisure-time activities
- Transport
- Public safety
- Social support
- Exposure to crime, violence, and social disorder
- Housing
- Language/literacy
- Access to mass media and emerging technologies
- Access to culture facilities.

The above list of social determinants is not exhaustive and the way they affect health in different countries may be context dependent. Much of the available evidence on the social determinants of health and the health effects of social interventions relate to more developed countries such as those found in Europe, North America, and Australasia. The evidence base underpinning our understanding of HPP is weaker for developing countries, which face different challenges in improving health and reducing health inequalities. However, as globalization continues, some of the health problems that have generally been associated with wealthier nations (for example, obesity) are increasingly becoming a problem for less developed countries, so evidence on the social determinants of health in developed countries may become more widely applicable.

A brief history of HPP

The idea that the health of the public can be affected, intentionally or otherwise, by the actions of planners or policy-makers across a range of sectors is of course not unique to the twentieth century. For example, in the mid nineteenth century, Edwin Chadwick made clear the link between poor living standards and high mortality, drew on comparative national and international data, and argued the case for government action. This helped create the conditions that led to the British Public Health Act of 1848, which resulted in improvements in sanitation, sewerage, and public administration, and can be seen as an early example of research informing an inter-sectoral health strategy.

The term 'Healthy Public Policy' itself can be traced to the 1970s and 1980s, when social researchers became increasingly critical of the narrow focus of much public health research at that time, which seemed to concentrate on disease processes and health care interventions, rather than the wider social and physical environment. The 1978 WHO Declaration of Alma-Ata (WHO, 1978) formally acknowledged the importance of inter-sectoral action for health. Nancy Milo's book *Promoting Health through Public Policy* (Milo, 1981) is often heralded as an important milestone in advocating the potential of public policy as a tool for health promotion. In 1986, the WHO adopted the Ottawa Charter, which called on countries to use multi-sectoral policy to promote health (WHO, 1986).

Nearly 20 years later, in 2005, the Bangkok Charter emphasized again that health is the business of all sectors: 'Responsibility to address the determinants of health rests with the whole of government, and depends upon actions by many sectors as well as the health sector' (WHO, 2005). The WHO Commission on Social Determinants of Health reiterated this point in 2008 (WHO, 2008). A number of countries have now adopted inter-sectoral approaches to public health, often under the banner of 'Health in All Policies'. These include Australia, Canada, USA, Finland, France, and Thailand.

The focus of Healthy Public Policy: upstream and downstream factors

A metaphor sometimes used in public health circles depicts illness as a river that people find themselves 'pushed into' by adverse socio-economic conditions. They then float down the river until, if they are lucky, the health service intervenes and pulls them out. The health service clearly performs a vital role in this (admittedly simplistic) scene but the public health response is to look further up the river and address those circumstances that make people fall in to begin with: prevention being preferred to cure. Many of the circumstances that might push people towards well-being on the one hand and ill health on the other operate on a macro or population level and are sometimes termed 'upstream'. These are the social determinants of health. Environments, be they legal, political, economic, physical or social, are considered to be 'upstream' and attempts to modify these environments to improve health are sometimes called 'social', 'structural' or 'upstream' health interventions (Dahlgren and Whitehead, 2006).

Health is also determined by individual-level factors, centring on people's lifestyle choices, behaviours, and personal coping strategies. Attempts to modify these individual-level determinants are sometimes referred to as 'downstream', 'lifestyle' or 'behavioural change' interventions (Dahlgren and Whitehead, 2006). These, too, may have non-health sector settings, such as in schools or workplaces. Some lifestyle interventions have been shown to be effective, but others less so – perhaps, so the argument goes, because individual choices and behaviours cannot be addressed effectively without also modifying the upstream environmental factors that shape them.

Some political ideologies favour these 'downstream' approaches over 'upstream' ones due to a preference for policies that emphasize individual choice and a mistrust of large-scale state intervention. In the UK, the political ideology 'Thatcherism', popular in the 1980s, seemed to embody these views, while in the USA and elsewhere neo-liberal conservatism occupies a similar ideological space. However, left-wing governments have also been accused of 'lifestyle drift': that is, an initial enthusiasm and rhetoric focused on tackling upstream determinants of poor health that is subsequently abandoned in favour of more individualist approaches as part of a general watering down of more radical policies (Popay *et al.*, 2010).

The focus of Healthy Public Policy: improving population health or reducing health inequalities

The debate over the relative merits of upstream and downstream approaches to public health permeates discussions of HPP but it is not the only dilemma faced within this area of policy. More fundamental still is the question of what the overall goal of HPP should be. The social determinants of health are often discussed in relation to two related but distinct public health goals: population health improvement and reductions in inequalities in health (Graham, 2007). Sometimes health policy discussions conflate these concepts but it is important to recognize that they can be very different. In fact, population health improvement and reductions in health inequalities require distinct public health strategies that at times can be mutually exclusive and therefore involve prioritizing one goal over the other. Macintyre has pointed out that the decision about which goal to pursue cannot be based on evidence alone but also depends on the decision-makers' values (Macintyre, 2007).

Public health policy in many countries is increasingly concerned with health inequalities. While population health is often improving, there are entrenched and systematic differences in health outcomes between population sub-groups and a social gradient in health whereby the lower a person's social position, the worse his or her health (Marmot *et al.*, 2010). The reasons for these health inequalities are widely accepted to lie predominantly 'upstream' rather than 'downstream'. Healthy Public Policy could therefore potentially reduce health inequalities by tackling issues such as those described below (Wilkinson and Marmot, 2003; Marmot *et al.*, 2010).

- *Social exclusion*: results from discrimination, stigmatization, hostility, poverty, and unemployment. These processes can be mutually reinforcing, contributing to 'disadvantage' by preventing equal access to education, training, services, and citizenship activities.

- *Working conditions*: in general, having a job is better for health than having no job. But the social organization of work, job security, management styles, and social relationships in the workplace all tend to be patterned so that jobs with lower social status tend to have less favourable working conditions.
- *Social support*: helps give people the emotional and practical resources they need. Isolation is associated with low well-being and disadvantage.
- *Access to commodities associated with healthy or less healthy lifestyles*: the price, marketing, and local availability of commodities such as alcohol, tobacco, and foods that are associated with healthy or less healthy diet. The geographic distribution of such commodities can be socially patterned.
- *Housing*: ensuring homes are of an adequate size, not too expensive to heat, free from damp, pollutants and structural problems, as well as places where people feel safe, happy and in control. Housing markets enable those with higher incomes to afford better quality homes in more desirable neighbourhoods.
- *Transport*: healthy transport means less driving and more walking and cycling, backed up by better public transport.

Bambra *et al.* (2011) have pointed out that public health reports on tackling health inequalities commissioned by successive UK governments over three decades present recommendations covering social determinants that include a focus on: early years and young people; education, training, and employment opportunities; working conditions; poverty and the distribution of wealth/resources; housing; transport; services infrastructure and amenities (from both public and private sectors). During this 30 year period there has, however, been relatively little progress in reducing health inequalities. Explanations for this include the feasibility and effectiveness of the recommendations, and whether decision-makers have lacked the political will to deliver sufficiently radical strategies (Mackenbach, 2012).

The unintended negative effects of public policies

One of the key concerns about public policy is the potential for unintended negative effects on health, and in particular the possibility that well-intentioned policies may unwittingly increase inequalities in health by having a greater impact on the better off. Health education is one often-cited example, It is argued that the generally better educated middle classes are likely to benefit more from the provision of health information to a population, and so provision of information in this way may actually risk increasing health inequalities (Wanless, 2004; Lorenc *et al.*, 2012).

Policies to control smoking are another example. Tobacco control policies in the UK since the 1970s have been accompanied by widening gaps between manual and non-manual socio-economic groups. It is therefore essential that interventions to prevent the uptake of smoking, or to promote smoking cessation, are effective among disadvantaged groups, and do not contribute to a continuing widening of inequalities (Thomas *et al.*, 2008).

Taxes on cigarettes are often seen as an important means of controlling smoking, but a government commissioned report on public health in the UK (Wanless, 2004) has examined how government could use taxes and subsidies more generally as levers to improve health. One example given by Wanless is the taxation of potentially unhealthy foods. Increasing the tax on foods with high levels of salt and fat might be used in an attempt to reduce their consumption. However, he warned that whether or not such benefits would materialize in practice depends on two factors. First, there is not usually a simple relationship between one type of food and health outcomes, so it is not clear that simply taxing fatty foods would lower obesity or reduce rates of coronary disease. Second, consumers and producers would find ways to avoid new taxes in ways that do not necessarily promote healthier behaviour. We know in the case of cigarettes that taxation often results in tobacco smuggling, so cheap cigarettes remain available.

As an alternative to taxes, subsidies can be used to promote health behaviours but these too can contribute to the creation of inequalities, as one example dealing with subsidizing gym use from the Wanless Report (2004) illustrates. Given the positive externalities associated with physical exercise, it could be argued that gyms should be subsidized. Although there is a case for government intervention to support physical activity, a simple gym subsidy is likely to be ineffective and inequitable because:

- Subsidizing gym fees, which are typically charged on a monthly basis and are not related to the amount of exercise undertaken, could encourage gym membership without actually encouraging exercise;
- Much of the subsidy would go to people who are already going to a gym or are likely to do so – the people who tend to be healthier; and
- Gym membership is more prevalent in the more healthy middle classes, and gyms are not found in all locations, so the subsidy will tend to assist certain healthier sections of society more, increasing health inequalities.

Such examples illustrate several of the characteristics of healthy public policies: they should contribute to the creation of environments which are protective of the health of individuals and communities but they should not inadvertently cause harm to the public's health nor should they contribute to the creation or exacerbation of existing health inequalities.

✏ Activity 5.2

Why might the twin public health goals of (1) overall population health improvement and (2) reducing health inequalities at times conflict and require different Healthy Public Policy strategies?

Feedback

The health problems of the most disadvantaged population sub-groups are notoriously complex and deeply embedded, which may particularly limit the effectiveness of policies and interventions designed to improve their health. In some circumstances, targeting more advantaged sub-groups may produce more aggregate health gain at relatively less cost. Targeting disadvantaged populations may produce less, and more costly, aggregate health gain but this gain will be focused where the need is greatest (Macintyre, 2007).

To reduce health inequalities, public health policies must ensure that resource allocation and the distribution of services take account of unequal levels of need. Such policies may exclusively target disadvantaged groups or they may provide universal coverage but with resource allocation and intervention delivery proportionally weighted to reflect a gradient of need, an approach known as 'proportionate universalism'

(Marmot *et al.*, 2010). Interventions will widen health inequalities if exposure, uptake, and effects turn out to be socially patterned in ways that most benefit already advantaged groups. A recent scoping of the literature on interventions that generate inequalities concluded that downstream interventions do not appear to reduce inequalities, and may increase them, citing evidence from media campaigns and workplace smoking bans as examples (Lorenc *et al.*, 2012).

Intervention inequalities may also occur if disadvantaged sub-groups experience unintended adverse impacts. For example, attempts to reduce smoking by raising tobacco prices can be said to have a disproportionately greater impact on people with the least disposable income. This may explain why price controls appear to have been effective in reducing tobacco-related health inequalities, but it raises the question of whether such policies add to the financial disadvantages experienced by low-income households where the prevalence of smoking tends to be higher (Thomas *et al.*, 2008).

Delivering HPP

In addition to questions about the aims of HPP, there are practical challenges that can impede its successful delivery. First, there are challenges around knowledge and evidence. Non-health sector involvement in HPP may be hampered by a lack of understanding of public health issues within organizations. Furthermore, the availability of appropriate evidence that might inform HPP decision-making is often poor.

Second, there are challenges relating to the organizational support and structures that facilitate inter-sectoral working. Healthy Public Policy will often require high-level support across sectors with the enthusiasm of key individuals likely to make a crucial impact. It cannot be assumed that the aims and goals of the different sectors involved are always compatible and so there may be conflicts of interest.

The following sub-sections further explore these challenges and how they might be overcome.

Evidence to inform HPP

The first issue relating to evidence is how to identify those policies and interventions that are likely to have an effect on health and how to quantify these potential effects. Health impact assessment (HIA) has been advanced as an approach to help with these tasks. HIA developed from a concern that major public policies could have negative health effects. The importance of HIA has been emphasized in successive World Health Organization (WHO) and European Union (EU) policy documents and is currently being used in countries around the world.

Broadly, HIA involves two initial stages:

- *Screening* is a process by which policies, programmes or projects are assessed to determine whether they may have a health impact, and what type of impact. This may be done on the basis of expert knowledge and available evidence (Kemm and Parry, 2004).
- *Scoping* is a process by which further information is sought on the potential direct and indirect health effects of the proposed policy, and in which the methods, resources, participants, and the time-frame for the further HIA process are assessed.

These stages will reveal whether there is a need for further work, which could include a *rapid health impact appraisal*, which is a systematic assessment by a number of experts, decision-makers, and representatives of the health impacts of a proposed policy or intervention. This in turn may lead to a more in-depth *health impact analysis* or, where an in-depth analysis is not possible, a *health impact review*, which aims to estimate the most significant health impacts of a particular activity based on the available evidence as well as expert consultations.

Numerous HIAs have now been published, and the methods are subject to constant revision (for example, Kemm and Parry, 2004). Whether HIA really succeeds in achieving Healthy Public Policy in practice may be difficult to determine. The strength and consistency of the available evidence varies greatly by subject area and the resources committed to HIA can be inadequate (Thomson, 2008). This variability of evidence suggests that the findings of some HIAs are likely to be more valid than others. Practitioners need to be aware of this variability, utilizing the *best available evidence* while understanding the limitations of that evidence.

The second issue relating to evidence concerns the effectiveness of HPP. Since the 1990s, commentators have criticized public health researchers for failing to conduct evaluations of policy-relevant interventions that could provide decision-makers with robust evidence of what works, who it works for, and in what circumstances (Petticrew *et al.*, 2004). This problem of insufficient evidence persists. Bambra *et al.* (2010) reported on an attempt to comprehensively identify systematic reviews addressing the effects on health and health inequalities of interventions targeting the social determinants of health in developed countries. Only 30 systematic reviews of upstream interventions were identified across a wide range of policy areas that included housing, transport, workplace, unemployment, welfare, agriculture, food, water, and sanitation. Furthermore, only three of these reviews presented evidence on how interventions differentially affected population sub-groups. Even in those three reviews, the evidence identified was weak (Bambra *et al.*, 2010).

This lack of evidence means in reality that HPP must frequently be developed in the absence of clear evidence regarding *what works, for whom and in what context* (Pawson and Tilley, 1997). The lack of evidence is not an excuse for political inaction, but it does highlight the importance of ensuring that future interventions are well evaluated and that evidence of impacts on different social groups are explored.

Inter-sectoral working

While the evidence base may be under-developed, there remains scope for different sectors to combine and create innovative HPP strategies, providing they can achieve effective working partnerships. However, in practice stakeholders may not support this approach equally. HPP can be criticized for justifying a kind of 'health imperialism', where people from the health sector attempt to put their concerns at the top of all other sectors' agendas. Underlying this criticism are questions of values and practical politics.

In terms of values, people tend to agree that public health is important but opinions differ about the specific instances where it should be considered the main priority. As is often the case in politics, there can be a difference between rhetoric and practice regarding the relative importance given to health concerns in other sectors. In a Dutch study (De Leeuw and Clavier, 2011), stakeholders from professional associations, consumer groups, researchers, non-governmental organizations, political parties, ministers, and advisory councils were consulted in connection with a parliamentary resolution advancing

HPP. While the researchers found that stakeholders were generally willing to express the view that HPP was a good idea in principle, this apparent approval did not lead to tangible activities or outputs. In fact, the researchers claimed that the majority of stakeholders, including many who were particularly influential, 'fought a silent battle of attrition and benevolent dissociation' that led to the resolution's failure to obtain sufficient parliamentary support (De Leeuw and Clavier, 2011: ii240).

A key part of the Health in All Policies agenda is to develop practical ways of tackling some of the barriers that, as in the case above, impede inter-sectoral action. Stakeholders are advised to seek 'win–win solutions': that is, actions that benefit the interests of all parties (Freiler *et al.*, 2013). So, for example, encouraging active modes of travel such as walking and cycling rather than reliance on cars serves public health interests, because physical activity benefits health, but could also potentially help transport managers reduce traffic congestion with (in theory) economic benefits resulting from more efficient transportation networks. The win–win approach depends on identifying those interventions that serve multiple interests. It is also a rhetorical device: a means of presenting health policies and interventions in a way that will appeal to multi-sectoral partners.

Healthy Public Policy can also be advanced by improving understanding about health issues within different sectors (Freiler *et al.*, 2013). This includes building capacity through workshops, training, secondments, and awareness-raising. Enlisting key individuals from different sectors who have a knowledge and interest in health is important, but the Health in All Policies approach also emphasizes the need to embed capacity within institutional structures, and provide non-health sectors with access to health expertise. For example, a reform of the English National Health Service (NHS) in 2013 led to its public health practitioners being transferred from the NHS to local authorities so that they would be institutionally closer to decision-makers responsible for many of those local services that are related to social determinants of health, such as schools, transport networks, town planning, and licensing of alcohol outlets.

Conflicts of interests

Win–win solutions are not always possible. This chapter has already described how, within public health, the competing goals of health improvement and health inequality reduction are not always reconcilable. Un-reconcilable goals are also likely between sectors: indeed, public health advocates have at times aligned themselves against specific interests within non-health sectors over issues such as finance and economic policy, transport, welfare, and working conditions. Such conflicts are likely to multiply if HPP extends beyond the public sector and into the third and private sectors. For instance, it is impossible to imagine a win–win solution that could reconcile the interests of public health and the tobacco industry. When conflicts of interest arise, it can be helpful to identify other allies who may stand to benefit from HPP. For example, in the case of tobacco, insurance companies and unions representing workers exposed to high levels of secondary tobacco smoke have supported proposals for smoke-free workplaces.

Even when goals can be aligned, there are still likely to be compromises on both sides. A recurring problem relates to budgeting. One potential risk from HPP is that finite public health resources may become spread more thinly as a result of inter-sectoral action. For example, although public health budgets in the UK health reforms were ring-fenced following the transfer to local authorities in 2013, there remains a fear that money once used for core public health functions within the health service may eventually be re-allocated into a range of different local authority budgets without proper consideration of the costs and benefits of such a transfer (Green, 2013).

Both technical expertise and diplomacy are required to sustain relationships between sectors, negotiate trade-offs, and agree on resource allocations. To bridge different understandings of a problem and align vested interests, a sound knowledge of the main stakeholders' perspectives can be crucial. Krech (2011) suggests that this explains why negotiations for some of the major international health agreements have been led by experienced diplomats rather than health experts.

How HPP has been used in practice

This section of the chapter provides some real-life examples of how HPP has been used or promoted at different policy levels.

HPP at an international level

The European Union Common Agricultural Policy (CAP) exemplifies how international policy can affect public health. The CAP was established to deal with food shortages after the Second World War by maintaining prices for fruit and vegetables and protecting farmers from competition by taxing imports. The EC has since become the focal point for public health advocates seeking to achieve Healthy Public Policy goals through the CAP. This has at times meant challenging CAP policies considered to be detrimental to public health goals. For instance, in 2012, the European Public Health and Agriculture Consortium (EPHAC) criticized an agreement on reforming the CAP as a missed opportunity for putting better nutrition for all at the centre of farming and food systems. On a positive note, EPHAC successfully advocated for the provision of free fruit for European school children and for an international agreement not to re-introduce direct support to tobacco growing (EPHAC, 2013).

HPP at national and regional levels

The North Karelia Project was launched in Finland in 1972 with the aim of reducing coronary heart disease in the Finnish region of North Karelia (Puska et al., 2009). The project resulted in significant reductions in cardiovascular disease mortality through joint action to improve community health, working with community organizations, farmers, and schools. In 2001, Finland developed the 'Health 2015' cooperation programme that seeks to promote health and healthy lifestyles, as well as reducing health inequalities, through a framework for inter-sectoral health promotion.

Some national and regional governments have adopted health impact assessments (HIAs) as a tool for advancing HPP. For example, following the reform of Thailand's National Health System in 2000, HIAs were made mandatory for all levels of government and have been used to tackle health problems caused by environmental hazards linked to pesticides, coal-fired plants, and other sources of pollution (Phoolcharoen et al., 2003).

Created in 2010, California's Health in All Policies Task Force is a statewide effort to bring together 19 different state agencies and departments to develop health improvement strategies. The 2010 'Health in All Policies Task Force Report to the Strategic Growth Council' emphasized the need for health consequences to be considered during policy recommendations and made specific recommendations regarding state policy on transport, housing, affordable healthy food, safe neighborhoods, and green space (Health in All Policies Task Force, 2010).

HPP at a local level

De Leeuw and Clavier (2011) argue that local government presents particularly favourable conditions for HPP, as local policy processes are less sector-based, involve adaptive leadership and more flexible partnership arrangements. The Healthy Cities Movement is often cited as a model for encouraging inter-sectoral action to plan for health at a local level (Lipp *et al.*, 2012).

However, there are also barriers to HPP at a local level. In a study of local authorities in London in the UK, Martineau *et al.* (2013) have outlined some of the challenges. They include managing competing interests among local stakeholders (including the electorate), rigid regulatory frameworks, relatively modest resources, and the frequent need to adapt to changing priorities and regulations affecting partners in other sectors. The study used the licensing of alcohol sales as an example of how such constraints operate in practice. Although public health practitioners are included in local license granting bodies, they must work within existing legal frameworks that prioritize public order and safety over long-term health risks. Local authorities also face legal challenges from well-resourced multinational businesses wishing to sell alcohol in their areas. Public health practitioners can, however, make the case for area-wide restrictions on new licensing and encourage alcohol outlets to engage in voluntary initiatives to reduce alcohol consumption. The public health practitioners who participated in the study advanced their case through good knowledge of the law, effective negotiations with other stakeholders, and by developing local evidence to support their case. So there are ways of promoting a public health agenda locally but they require public health practitioners to work imaginatively within a framework and with partners whose priorities are not precisely aligned with their own (Martineau *et al.*, 2013, Phillips and Green, 2015).

Summary

This chapter has outlined some of the ways in which HPP can be developed to advance public health goals by modifying the social determinants of health. It has also considered some of the barriers to HPP, such as competing understandings and lack of clarity regarding the aims of HPP; a lack of evidence on the health effects (especially effects on health inequalities) of interventions that modify social determinants of health; and divisions and conflicts of interests that occur at all policy levels and between sectors. Such barriers can be deeply embedded and complex, but there are distinct ways in which the public health community can take action to overcome them. The aims of HPP can be clarified with respect to population health improvement or reductions in health inequalities. Further research into the effects of interventions relevant to HPP can improve the evidence base to inform decision-making. Divisions between sectors and departments can be bridged through mutually beneficial stakeholder alliances supported by personal and structural links. Policies and structures that exacerbate health inequalities can be identified, challenged, and reformed. Through such actions, Healthy Public Policy should play a leading role in furthering long-term public health goals by bringing improvements and greater equity to the social determinants of health.

References

Bambra, C., Gibson M., Sowden, A., Wright, K., Whitehead, M. and Petticrew, M. (2010) Tackling the wider social determinants of health and health inequalities: evidence from systematic reviews, *Journal of Epidemiology and Community Health*, 64: 284–9.

Bambra, C., Smith, K.E., Garthwaite, K., Joyce, K. and Hunter, D. (2011) A labour of Sisyphus? Public policy and health inequalities research from the Black and Acheson Reports to the Marmot Review, *Journal of Epidemiology and Community Health*, 65: 399–406.

Dahlgren, G. and Whitehead, M. (2006) *Levelling Up (Part 2): A Discussion Paper on European Strategies for Tackling Social Inequities in Health*. Geneva: WHO Regional Office for Europe [http://www.who.int/social_determinants/resources/leveling_up_part2.pdf].

De Leeuw, E. and Clavier, C. (2011) Healthy public in all policies, *Health Promotion International*, 26 (suppl. 2): ii237–ii244.

European Public Health and Agriculture Consortium (EPHAC) (2013) Lost opportunity to recognise public health and nutrition dimension of European farming and rural development policy (Media Statement). Brussels: EPHAC.

Freiler, A., Muntaner, C. and Shankardass, K. (2013) Glossary for the implementation of Health in All Policies (HiAP), *Journal of Epidemiology and Community Health*, 67: 1068–72.

Graham, H. (2007) *Unequal Lives: Health and Socioeconomic Inequalities*. Buckingham: Open University Press.

Green, J. (2013) *Public Health and Local Government: Challenges and Possibilities*. CEIPS Discussion Paper #2013-01. Melbourne, VIC: Centre of Excellence in Intervention and Prevention Science.

Health in All Policies Task Force (2010) *Report to the Strategic Growth Council: Executive Summary*. Sacramento, CA: HiAP Task Force [http://sgc.ca.gov/docs/HiAP_Task_Force_Executive_Summary_Dec_2010.pdf].

Kemm, J. and Parry, J. (2004) What is HIA? Health impact assessment, in J. Kemm, J. Parry and S. Palmer (eds.) *Health Impact Assessment*. Oxford: Oxford University Press.

Krech, R. (2011) Healthy public policies: looking ahead, *Health Promotion International*, 26 (suppl. 2): ii268–ii272.

Lipp, A., Winters, T. and de Leeuw, E. (2012) Evaluation of partnership working in cities in phase IV of the WHO Healthy Cities Network, *Journal of Urban Health*, 90 (suppl. 1): 37–51.

Lorenc, T., Petticrew, M., Welch, V. and Tugwell, P. (2012) What types of interventions generate inequalities? Evidence from systematic reviews, *Journal of Epidemiology and Community Health*, 67: 190–3.

Macintyre, S. (2007) *Inequalities in Health in Scotland: What are they and what can we do about them?* Occasional Paper #17. Glasgow: MRC Social and Public Health Sciences Unit.

Mackenbach, J.P. (2012) The persistence of health inequalities in modern welfare states: the explanation of a paradox, *Social Science and Medicine*, 75: 761–9.

Marmot, M., Allen, J., Goldblatt, P., Boyce, T., Mcneish, D., Grady, M. *et al.* (2010) *Fair Society, Healthy Lives: The Marmot Review – Strategic Review of Health Inequalities in England Post 2010*. London: University College London.

Martineau, F.P., Graff, H., Mitchell, C. and Lock, K. (2013) Responsibility without legal authority? Tackling alcohol-related health harms through licensing and planning policy in local government, *Journal of Public Health*, 36 (3): 435–42.

Milo, N. (1981) *Promoting Health through Public Policy*. Philadelphia, PA: Davis.

Pawson, R. and Tilley, N. (1997) *Realistic Evaluation*. London: Sage.

Petticrew, M., Whitehead, M., Macintyre, S., Graham, H. and Egan, M. (2004) Evidence for public health policy on inequalities: 1. The reality according to policymakers, *Journal of Epidemiology and Community Health*, 58: 811–16.

Phillips, G. and Green, J. (2015) Working for the public health: politics, localism and epistemologies of practice, *Sociology of Health and Illness*, 37 (3).

Phoolcharoen, W., Sukkumnoed, D. and Kessomboon, P. (2003) Development of health impact assessment in Thailand: recent experiences and challenges, *Bulletin of the World Health Organization*, 81: 465–7.

Popay, J., Whitehead, M. and Hunter, D. (2010) Injustice is killing people on a large scale – but what is to be done about it?, *Journal of Public Health*, 32: 148–9.

Puska, P., Vartiainen, E., Laatikainen, T., Jousilahti, P. and Paavola, M. (eds.) (2009) *The North Karelia Project: From North Karelia to National Action*. Helsinki: National Institute for Health and Welfare.

Thomas, S., Fayter, D., Misso, K., Ogilvie, D., Petticrew, M., Sowden, A. *et al.* (2008) Population tobacco control interventions and their effects on social inequalities in smoking: systematic review, *Tobacco Control*, 17: 230–7.

Thomson, H. (2008) HIA forecast: cloudy with sunny spells later? (Viewpoint), *European Journal of Public Health*, 18: 436–8.

Wanless, D. (2004) *Securing Good Health for the Whole Population: Final Report*. London: HMSO [http://webarchive.nationalarchives.gov.uk/+/http:/www.hm-treasury.gov.uk/media/D/3/Wanless04_summary.pdf].

Wilkinson, R. and Marmot, M. (2003) *Social determinants of Health: The Solid Facts*, 2nd edn. Geneva: WHO.

World Health Organization (WHO) (1978) *Declaration of Alma-Ata*. Geneva: WHO [http://www.who.int/publications/almaata_declaration_en.pdf].

World Health Organization (WHO) (1986) *Ottawa Charter for Health Promotion*. Geneva: WHO [http://www.who.int/healthpromotion/conferences/previous/ottawa/en/].

World Health Organization (WHO) (2005) *Bangkok Charter for Health Promotion*. Geneva: WHO [http:www.who.int/healthpromotion/conferences/6gchp/pr_050829_%20BCHP.pdf].

World Health Organization (WHO) (2008) *Closing the Gap in a Generation: Health Equity through Action on the Social Determinants of Health*. Final Report of the Commission on Social Determinants of Health. Geneva: WHO.

6 Advocacy for health

James Chauvin and Heather Yeatman

Overview

This chapter starts by describing advocacy for health – a deliberate pro-activist process that uses strategic actions to influence others to shift opinion, initiate positive change, counter misinformation, and address underlying factors that affect human health. The chapter goes on to provide several frameworks that have been developed to guide advocacy for health. It then explores the development of advocacy for health and the role played by public health associations. It provides practical examples of how to undertake advocacy for health using case studies. Finally, the chapter identifies advocacy enablers and barriers.

Learning objectives

After reading this chapter, you will be able to:

- define advocacy for health
- describe a range of advocacy initiatives undertaken to achieve improvements in public health outcomes
- analyse the use of advocacy for different settings or for different health policy outcomes
- identify the enabling factors and challenges for advocacy
- identify ways in which professionals, associations, and organizations can collaborate with civil society to advocate for healthy policies and best practice for health

Key terms

Advocacy: A catch-all word for the set of skills used to create a shift in public opinion and mobilize the necessary resources and forces to support an issue, policy or constituency.

Civil society voice: Proactive communication by the non-governmental sector (communities, NGOs, professional associations) to influence thinking and action within political space for the public good.

Healthy Public Policy: A protocol for the common good that seeks to create a supportive environment across all areas of government jurisdiction, enabling people to live healthy lives, incorporating public accountability by government for health and health equity impact as a result of all policies enacted.

Lobbying: A form of advocacy which, through proactive and direct action, usually with remuneration or financial self-interest, applies pressure and influence on public officials and governments' formulation of policies and programmes.

What is advocacy for health?

Advocacy has been defined as 'a catch-all word for the set of skills used to create a shift in public opinion and mobilize the necessary resources and forces to support an issue, policy, or constituency . . . advocacy seeks to increase the power of people and groups and to make institutions more responsive to human needs. It attempts to enlarge the range of choices that people can have by increasing their power to define problems and solutions and participate in the broader social and policy arena' (Wallack et al., 1993: 27–8).

Although the Ottawa Charter for Health Promotion identified advocacy for health as a core health promotion strategy (WHO, 1986), it could be considered one of the least understood and most poorly explored aspects of health promotion. This may be because 'engaging in public health advocacy acknowledges the explicitly political aspects of public health, and the importance of addressing social determinants of health as a key component of a strategy for improving the health of populations' (Alberta Health Services, 2009: 1).

Advocacy for health is a deliberate pro-activist process that uses strategic actions to influence others for a variety of purposes, be it at the level of the individual (for example, personal behaviours affecting health) or population (for example, systemic, biomedical, and non-biomedical determinants affecting the health of communities and nations) (Canadian Public Health Association, 2010). As Chapman (2004: 361) points out, advocacy 'is often carried out in the face of opposition'. In addition, 'advocacy . . . recognizes the dynamic interplay of a myriad of factors and influences which often lie well beyond the reach of the [advocate's] desire for control' (Chapman, 2001: 1226).

The World Health Organization (1995) described advocacy for health as a 'combination of individual and social actions designed to gain political commitment, policy support, social acceptance and systems support for a particular health goal or programme'.

Advocacy for health goes beyond increasing awareness and educating people about an issue. It is a means to an end, which seeks to:

- enable people and communities to gain access to, and a voice in, the decision-making process of relevant institutions and organizations, be they governmental or non-governmental, for-profit or not-for-profit;
- change the power relationships between these institutions and the people affected by their decisions, thereby potentially changing the institutions themselves;
- improve the overall health of a population and bring a clear improvement in people's lives;
- pursue an ethical course of action that addresses social justice and health equity (Carlisle, 2000).

Advocacy creates the conditions for social change. As expressed by Avery and Bashir (2003: 1209), the biggest reward of advocacy 'is creating shoulders for others to stand on'.

Advocacy for health activities are not confined to any single location or setting. As Bassett (2003: 1204) puts it, '[Public] health takes place in boardrooms, on street corners, in our homes, and in the legislature. So, too, does [public] health advocacy.'

Although the terms 'advocacy' and 'lobbying' are sometimes used interchangeably, many consider that they are not the same (United States Senate, 1995; Minister of Justice, 2006; Moore, 2011; Public Health Agency of Canada, undated). Lobbying can be considered as one form of advocacy with a financial reward or another type of incentive that is directed to public officials in a specific attempt to influence legislation, regulation or public policy (Connecticut Association of Nonprofits, 2003). Advocacy can refer to similar types of actions but is directed to a range of entities, including service providers, private and public organizations, communities, and individuals. Like lobbying, the outcome or outcomes sought through advocacy may be to change policy or regulation. Advocacy may also seek to bring about changes to service provision, limiting or expanding a company's activities or changes in personal opinions or behaviours, albeit for the public good rather than for personal or private gain.

Advocacy for health is a combination of art and science, which should be grounded in sound scientific and/or real-world evidence. As Chapman (2001: 1227) states, 'epidemiology is the bedrock on which advocacy should rest'. However, as he and others point out, the generation and communication of sound evidence alone are not sufficient preconditions to effective advocacy. Effective advocacy demands a blend of skills and competencies, among which is an understanding of how decision-making systems work (be they government or non-government) and how the goals of the advocacy effort will interact with existing public and/or private sector priorities and concerns – in other words, a strong dash of political science. The successful advocate also needs to know how to frame and deliver the argument – which entails well-honed communications skills. A health advocate cannot be risk-adverse. In most cases, although lessons can be learned and applied from others' experiences, health advocates often move forward by instinct and by recognizing and being able to make the most of opportunities as they arise.

🖉 Activity 6.1

Identify a principal area for health advocacy in your location. Identify the aim and objectives of the advocacy and prepare a mapping of the political context that an advocacy effort on this issue might face.

Feedback

You may have identified a pressing health-related issue that requires a policy or regulatory action. You will then have defined the aim and objectives of the advocacy effort. You may also have prepared a grid listing the various stakeholders as potential allies or opponents, the degree to which you think they will engage on the issue, and the stance you think they will take on the issue. You may also have thought about how a shift in the focus of the advocacy objectives might affect stakeholders' positions (is there flexibility/is a compromise position possible?). You will also have started to map out the position of stakeholders and their reasons for these positions; and how you might approach each stakeholder in terms of convincing them to sign on as part of an alliance, or how you will deal with them as an opponent.

Getting organized for advocacy

There is no standard 'recipe book' for advocacy. There are, nonetheless, different ways to understand, plan for, and take health advocacy action. These processes will vary depending on the issue, who is involved, the level of preparedness, the opportunities that emerge, and the time that is available. Different authors and groups provide various frameworks to understand advocacy actions.

The US-based organization Program for Appropriate Technology for Health (PATH) developed a ten-step process for creating a policy advocacy strategy, many components of which align with systematic programme planning used in other areas of health promotion (PATH, 2013). Interestingly, the PATH approach appears to have an objective, almost dispassionate approach to selecting the issue to be the focus of advocacy, rather than starting with an issue that people or organizations feel strongly about as the impetus. This may be more common with advocacy-based organizations that need to weigh up the issues at which their limited resources should be directed. The PATH framework, described in Box 6.1, also primarily covers the planning phases in the preparation of an advocacy initiative.

A different approach is provided by the ten-step framework for public health advocacy developed by Moore et al. (2013), shown in Box 6.2. This approach is more a strategy for advocacy action. It starts with a higher level of engagement (Step 1: *establish a sense of urgency*), followed by almost a rallying call (*develop a change vision*) and various steps that indicate engagement (*communicating the vision for buy-in; never give up*) and action (*be opportunistic; generate short-term wins*). This framework is perhaps indicative of advocacy action for an issue about which individuals or agencies may be passionate. It also could be considered pertinent to advocacy that seeks to change policy.

Box 6.1 PATH's ten-step policy advocacy strategy

1. Identifying potential advocacy issues and choosing an advocacy issue
2. Identifying potential advocacy goals
3. Identifying decision-makers and influencers
4. Identifying decision-makers' key interests
5. Addressing opposition and overcoming obstacles
6. Taking inventory of advocacy assets and gaps and selecting advocacy partners
7. Developing objectives and a work plan
8. Crafting advocacy messages
9. Identifying advocacy messengers
10. Planning to measure success

Source: PATH (2013)

Box 6.2 Ten-step framework for public health advocacy

1. Establishing a sense of urgency
2. Creating the guiding coalition
3. Developing and maintaining influential relationships
4. Developing a change vision
5. Communicating the vision for buy-in
6. Empowering broad-based action
7. Be opportunistic
8. Generating short-term wins
9. Never give up
10. Incorporating changes into the culture

Source: Moore et al. (2013)

Another advocacy framework that is perhaps more relevant to individuals or community groups is a six-step approach developed by Conley-Wright and Jaffe (2014). This framework was developed by examining real-life child advocacy campaigns to provide support for parents who shared common challenges in meeting the special needs of their children. The steps outlined could be applied to other community-based issues, such as support for community vegetable gardens, or for vulnerable community members, such as appropriate services for homeless youths. The framework could be considered particularly relevant at the local level, when dealing with administrative processes or provision of services.

Box 6.3 Six-step approach to successful child advocacy

1. Knowing your issue
2. Conducting research
3. Preparing materials
4. Creating effective meetings
5. Conducting follow-up
6. Reinforcing positive outcomes

Source: Conley-Wright and Jaffe (2014)

✎ **Activity 6.2**

Return to the example you developed for Activity 6.1. Think about the three frameworks for advocacy described above: The PATH ten-step policy advocacy strategy (Box 6.1); the ten-step framework for public health advocacy developed by Moore and colleagues (Box 6.2); and the six-step approach developed by Conley-Wright and Jaffe (Box 6.3). Which one of these frameworks do you think you would use for your example?

Feedback

You may have reflected that the PATH framework involves identifying and selecting issues for advocacy, whereas the other two frameworks use an issue that has already been identified as their starting point. If your advocacy example is concerned with influencing national or organizational policy, you may find the ten-step framework of public health advocacy in Box 6.2 most useful. If your example involves influencing at a more local level, you may find the six steps in Box 6.3 more appropriate. There is no one correct answer. Each of these frameworks can be useful.

The development of health advocacy

One of the earliest examples of successful health advocacy occurred in mid-nineteenth-century England. In 1854, Dr. John Snow undertook what could be called the classic steps of advocacy:

*   He identified a problem – the sudden high number of cholera cases in the Soho area of London, a neighbourhood he served.

- He had a theory that the outbreak was related to the water system.
- He consulted with local residents of the neighbourhood of Soho about the source of their water.
- He conducted microscopic and chemical analysis of water samples from hand pumps in Soho and other neighbourhoods.
- He mapped the locations of cholera cases.
- He communicated the results in clear and simple means to the medical fraternity and municipal authorities, employing case reports and cartography (a dot map) to demonstrate the link between the quality of water at the public sources and cholera cases.
- He presented counter-arguments to his position.

His advocacy had the desired result: the local authorities had the handle of the Broad Street pump removed. This in turn had the desired effect: no recurrence of cholera cases in the neighbourhood; although Snow did acknowledge that the epidemic may have already been in decline before removal of the pump handle owing to people fleeing the area (Cameron and Jones, 1983).

Despite Snow's success in advocating for an action arising from a particular cholera epidemic, he failed to convince either the municipal authorities or his medical peers that future outbreaks could be controlled through improved sanitation, such as cleaning up cesspools and sewers. It would be several years before local health boards accepted the impact of water-borne diseases on health (Cameron and Jones, 1983).

Health advocacy blossomed in the early twentieth century. For example, a review of the minutes of the early meetings of the Board of Directors of the Canadian Public Health Association (CPHA), founded in 1910, and the archives of the *Canadian Journal of Public Health* revealed considerable advocacy efforts. The CPHA's early members advocated through a variety of means – including briefs, position papers, letters, meetings, and articles – for action to be taken by governmental authorities on a wide range of issues affecting human health. These issues included:

- Environmental health (water supply, sanitation, industrial effluent in rivers);
- The control of infectious diseases (tuberculosis, typhoid, smallpox, cholera, and syphilis);
- Health promotion (school-based health programmes, nutrition);
- Healthy urban development (green spaces, playgrounds for children); and
- The organization of the health care system (setting up of local health boards and provincial and federal ministries of health) (CPHA, 2010).

Around the same time, non-profit organizations were established in many countries to advocate for disease-specific issues. For example, the National Association for the Study and Prevention of Tuberculosis was founded in 1904. It later evolved into the American Lung Association. In 1913, the American Society for the Control of Cancer, which became the American Cancer Society, was established. Civil society organizations such as these were, and continue to be, important and ardent advocates for healthy public policy and practice.

Advocacy at the national level: public health associations

Public health associations (PHAs) are non-governmental, politically independent and authoritative voices dedicated to promote and protect the public's health. In some countries, they are its only voice. They play an important role in advocacy for health. This is, for many public health associations, their prime directive.

The advocacy contributions and influence of national PHAs are far reaching. Several have played leadership roles in the ongoing fight for tobacco control (Public Health Association of Australia, 2011). Others have focused their advocacy efforts on the prevention and control of both infectious and non-communicable diseases or on the quality of – and access to – essential public health services, such as immunization and maternal-newborn and child health services. Some PHAs have advocated for a social determinants of health approach to achieve better and more equitable health outcomes. Still others have championed politically sensitive causes, such as the prevention and treatment of HIV and AIDS, and have gained hard-won advances in access to essential medicines, to clean needle and syringe programmes, and to treatment protocols, including alternative pharmacotherapies for dependent drug users (Canadian Public Health Association, 2011).

Advocacy at the community level: grass roots advocacy

Health advocacy is not restricted to professional and highly visible and well-established organizations. There are many examples of effective grass-roots-generated health advocacy actions. The Treatment Action Campaign (TAC) was launched in 1998 in Capetown, South Africa by a handful of activists protesting about the lack of access to antiretroviral (ARV) therapies to all people in South Africa. Through a series of bold actions and well-planned and focused advocacy efforts (including taking the Government of South Africa to court), TAC succeeded in not only changing attitudes about HIV and ARV therapy among national political leaders, but also in increasing access to affordable ARV therapy to all who need it, including pregnant women as a preventive measure for mother-to-child transmission of HIV (TAC, 2003–2014).

Another example of a community-based grass-roots advocacy movement, and one that has evolved into a global campaign, centres around opposition to hydraulic fracking (Food & Water Watch, 2014). Fracking is a controversial technique to extract natural gas and oil from shale rock. Americans Against Fracking is one of several grass-roots organizations formed to oppose fracking, citing occupational health and safety concerns for those employed in the industry, as well as community environmental health concerns that include surface and underground water contamination, airborne pollution, toxic waste, and increased heavy industry-related traffic. Although the campaigns have not stopped hydraulic fracking, they have resulted in delaying extraction pending further research into health and ecosystem impacts in some countries and tighter regulations in others.

Using advocacy in practice: lessons from case studies

The following case studies highlight the advocacy efforts of several national PHAs. The first case study illustrates the ways and means that the Public Health Association of Australia (PHAA) adopted to address environmental issues as part of advocacy for food and nutrition policy. The second describes the efforts and achievements of three PHAs in Africa with respect to smoke-free workplaces and health facilities. The third case study presents the advocacy campaign by parents of young people with special needs in the USA. Although the types of advocacy are specific to these three case studies, the principles and lessons learned are applicable to other organizations, situations, and sectors.

Case study 6.1: Environmental issues as part of food and nutrition policy in Australia (Moore *et al.*, 2013)

Context of the advocacy actions

The Public Health Association of Australia (PHAA) was frustrated with the lack of a holistic food and nutrition policy at the national level. With the assistance of a variety of stakeholders, the PHAA developed a policy framework, *A Future for Food*, with the aim to influence government in their impending review of the National Dietary Guidelines and to pressure the government to develop a national food and nutrition policy (PHAA, 2009). Not only did this document – and a subsequent, updated document (Public Health Association of Australia, 2012) – form the basis of much media attention, it also provided a policy document for other organizations to use and formed the basis of later submissions and commentary while government policy activities were underway.

What was the role of evidence?

The advocacy document was based on the latest scientific evidence. This was critically important to the advocacy process, as the veracity of the position and statements made by the PHAA were closely scrutinized. In addition, as the evidence base had been well developed, it allowed the PHAA and other organizations to quickly respond to political and industry points of contention.

What were the main advocacy actions?

The main advocacy action was the development of the *Future for Food* documents. These formed the basis of all other actions, and provided a common vision for a range of organizations to use. Other actions included:

*   A national workshop and major literature review to inform the *Food for Future* documents;
*   Work with a number of other health-focused organizations;
*   Providing the *Food for Future* documents, in hard copy and often in person, to all members of parliament with a connection to the food system;
*   Extensive work with media to raise awareness of the issues using the *Food for Future* documents, as well as to forge positive relations with the media to support future advocacy actions;
*   Meetings with key individuals in partner organizations to ensure all were using the same messages.

What was the advocacy outcome?

Policy progress was achieved in two areas. The review of the Australian Dietary Guidelines for the first time included active debate on the environmental sustainability issues related to food and subsequently included considerations of these issues in an appendix to the official government document (National Health and Medical Research Council, 2013). When developing a national food plan, the Australian government also actively deliberated on the relationships between the food system and health. However, in the end nutrition and health issues, while mentioned, were not directly incorporated (Department of Agriculture, Fisheries and Forestry, 2013).

What were the main advocacy lessons learnt?

- Having a well-researched, well-presented policy document, when none had existed previously, provided a common platform for policy advocacy actions and messages;
- The document needed regular 'refreshing', not only to update scientific information, but also to provide a fresh 'look' to the advocacy activities;
- Such a document also provided a good resource for those within the organization and in other organizations who were new to policy advocacy, giving them confidence to speak about the matter in a number of forums.

Case study 6.2: Tobacco control in east and southern Africa

Context of the advocacy actions
Despite the ratification of the Framework Convention on Tobacco Control (FCTC), the development and application of policies and practices to reduce smoking prevalence and exposure to second-hand smoke were identified in 2012 as lacking or weak in some countries (Sekimpi *et al.*, 2012; Senkubuge *et al.*, 2012). The Tanzanian Public Health Association (TPHA), the Uganda National Association of Community and Occupational Health (UNACOH), and the Public Health Association of South Africa (PHASA) carried out an evidence-based advocacy campaign to promote the formulation and application of institutional policies for smoke-free workplaces and hospitals. Not only did their advocacy efforts have the desired effect, they also contributed to building these PHAs' advocacy capacity by forging links with organizations possessing advocacy experience and resources.

What was the role of evidence?
Obtaining the facts and building a solid evidence base about the absence or non-application of smoke-free policies and regulations was central to this exercise, as was the identification of resources and tools for health care providers to counsel patients who smoke (and their friends and family who visited them in hospital) to quit.

What were the main advocacy actions?
The main advocacy actions were recommendations to hospital administrators and senior medical staff about the importance of smoke-free health facilities and the ways and means to apply institutional smoke-free regulations. Other actions included:

- Literature reviews on the impact of institutional smoke-free health facilities to inform the advocacy document;
- Surveys of hospitals about the application of smoke-free regulations and of medical staff about their awareness of the health risk associated with second-hand smoke;
- Consultations with Ministry of Health representatives, hospital administrators and senior medical staff, and other health organizations;
- Media-related events about the advocacy efforts;
- Providing and training hospital staff about a smoke-free hospitals self-audit monitoring tool.

What was the advocacy outcome?

- Greater awareness among senior medical staff about the health risks associated with exposure to second-hand smoke;
- Some of the hospitals in each country adopted and applied a partial or full no-smoking policy.

What were the main advocacy lessons learnt?

- Dedicated staff with advocacy 'training' is essential;
- The lack of local evidence/documentation requires extra resources and time;
- Consultation with all stakeholders is important;
- Buy-in of hospital administrators and senior medical staff is important;
- Ministry of Health willingness to participate and buy-in to the effort is critical;
- Availability of tested resources and tools to facilitate the adoption of the proposed action by stakeholders is essential.

Case study 6.3: Advocacy by parents of young children with special needs (Conley-Wright and Taylor, 2014)

Context of the advocacy actions
Community members may seek to ensure that their and their family's needs are being met through advocacy actions. In the USA, legislation provides for appropriate services for young children with disabilities through the Individuals with Disabilities Act (IDEA). The legislation includes advocacy support and training for parents of children with disabilities, so they may act to ensure their child receives the services for which they are eligible. Through acting as advocates for their child, the parents become empowered themselves, which can assist them in dealing with the challenges they face as they look after their child's needs.

What was the role of evidence?
Parents were considered to be effective advocates for their child's needs because they know and understand their child's stage of development and can monitor modest changes in their child's needs on a daily basis. Parents are also constantly around, thus changes in service provision (for example, the unanticipated absence of a special needs service provider) can be quickly addressed.

What were the main advocacy actions?
Advocacy actions occurred in various settings – school, community, health services – and focused primarily on ensuring the children received the services they required and were eligible to receive. The advocacy training and support programme also provided networking opportunities for parents who otherwise would be living in fairly isolated circumstances and a mechanism by which information about availability of and changes to services could be readily disseminated.

What was the advocacy outcome?
The outcome of the advocacy actions extended beyond the individual child's or parent's needs. Parents themselves become better educated about the services

available for their child and their child's rights. In addition, the teachers and service providers who have contact with the child become better informed about the capacities (and limitations) of children with different disabilities, and their responsibilities under the legislation. Parents reported advocating with politicians to change legislation when flaws or inadequacies were identified. The advent of social media has also provided other avenues for dissemination of information about the needs of, and professionals' responsibilities towards, children with disabilities.

What were the main advocacy lessons learnt?

- The benefits of providing training and support to parents to enable them to be advocates;
- Some parents need ongoing support to sustain their advocacy actions;
- Advocacy skills can be shared with other parents through parent-to-parent mentoring;
- Empowerment of parents through their advocacy actions can serve to complement the role of professionals.

Advocacy 'enablers'

As Moore (undated: 36) observed, there is no 'silver bullet' or a single approach that guarantees success in advocacy and lobbying. In some instances, advocacy for health may be quite straightforward. In others, it may require considerable resources, time, persistence, and effort, owing to the complex web of structural, bureaucratic, political, and personal factors that characterize policy-making and decision-making (Shepherd, 2013). But, wherever it is undertaken, health advocacy requires thoughtful planning, method, and discipline. It cannot be carried out in a haphazard manner.

A prerequisite of good advocacy is a strong foundation (Independent Sector, 2012). The case studies cited above, along with the many documented analyses of advocacy efforts published in peer-reviewed journals, highlight several key factors as 'enablers' of advocacy (Chapman, 2001).

First, and arguably most important, is conducting a thorough pre-assessment or mapping of the advocacy issue context. Those engaged in advocacy need to understand who the key people are and how the decision-making system works. This mapping will help determine who are potential allies and who will potentially oppose the campaign. This might include conducting independent research to assess the views and opinions of the various stakeholders along with what positions and concessions they might be willing to accept or not accept.

Second, a key element is compiling a case based on solid evidence. The underlying facts and figures should be from independent, reliable, and credible sources. The arguments should be clearly presented, and could include if available an analysis of any counter-arguments. Understanding the 'other side of the coin' helps prepare a thorough understanding of the arguments in support of and opposed to the advocacy issue.

Third, a health advocate also needs to be able to recognize opportunities and take advantage of them. Knowing how and when to communicate, with messages tailored to specific target groups, is an important advocacy skill. As Shepherd (2013) notes, advocates spend a lot of time and effort assembling and analysing the evidence, but often they overlook or ignore the vital work of translating the research results into relevant and realistic policy options.

Fourth, advocacy requires good communication. Brief messaging is required. Short, clear, and concise briefing notes and advocacy that draws from personal stories have more appeal and impact. As Shepherd (2013) and others have observed, non-governmental advocates often lack effective communications skills, and their advocacy efforts suffer accordingly: 'The language used often slips into the imperative. The list of recommendations . . . is couched in terms of obligation . . . little thought [is] given to how the [proposed objectives] might be accomplished, or at what cost [and to whom]'.

Fifth, advocacy involves framing the issue effectively. Data and issues need to be communicated in ways that have resonance with the target audiences and are compelling in support of the particular issue (Alberta Health Services, 2009). Stone (1989) described this as telling a causal story, while others have referred to 'framing of an issue' (Chapman, 2001). The essence of framing is to describe the nature of the problem in a particular manner that identifies who is responsible and what (policy) action thus needs to occur. Existing policy areas need to be reframed so as to open up new possibilities with regard to health action. For example, problems associated with high alcohol consumption can be framed as a personal choice issue, with individuals being responsible for this action, and hence the policy required is one that is directed to individual behaviour change, either through education or penalties to stop particular actions such as driving while under the influence of alcohol. Alternatively, it can be framed as an access issue – alcohol is cheap to purchase and readily accessible, resulting in problematic drinking behaviours. In this framing of the issue, government could be considered responsible for limiting access to alcohol through imposing minimum prices for alcoholic drinks or regulating the opening hours of licensed venues.

Finally, good advocacy often requires developing solid relationships and alliances with other organizations. While obtaining consensus can be difficult, the sharing of resources will be of benefit to the advocacy effort. Diversity of opinion among coalition members is healthy – it helps form arguments and counter-arguments, and provides an opportunity to pilot-test the advocacy campaign activities beforehand. Creating strength in numbers can have the effect of counter-balancing the opposition's resources.

Barriers and challenges to advocacy

There are several identified barriers and challenges to successful advocacy actions. In response to an unpublished survey conducted by the World Federation of Public Health Associations (WFPHA) in 2011, member public health associations identified several issues of particular importance, including:

- Finding and generating the evidence base in resource-constrained settings;
- Lack of appropriate and adequate advocacy skills;
- Restrictions placed by governments on advocacy by NGOs (constraints on 'democratic space');
- Resistance of governments and corporations to listen and act in the public interest;
- Unequal resources to engage with advocacy and the power of opposing camps (WFPHA, 2011).

Another important challenge faced by advocates is the lack of methods and means to measure the impact of advocacy efforts. Assessing whether advocacy actually works is a relatively new field that requires overt attention. Webster et al. (2014) and others have pointed out that it is difficult to assess the impact of advocacy, to make a link between cause and effect, as advocacy on policy is rarely done in a controlled, closed environment. It is not simply a matter of counting the outputs (for example, the number of meetings held, the number of pamphlets printed and distributed, the number of 'hits' on an advocacy-dedicated website). Chapman (2001) has suggested that more qualitative approaches may be useful. He suggested using a critical path framework (changing perceptions of key gatekeepers including the public and media), discourse analysis of media reporting and commentary as means of mapping changing opinions and how the issue is framed; and critical reflective accounts of the advocacy process written by those who were involved. This may be helpful in illuminating a particular type of advocacy, when media or public opinion is part of either the advocacy process or a desired outcome. However, researching advocacy actions and impacts at local levels or within organizations or discrete sectors is likely to require different approaches.

Activity 6.3

Conduct a web-based search of evaluations or journal articles on health advocacy-related issues. Select at least two examples. Prepare a list of enabling factors and barriers that affected the health advocacy efforts and compare/contrast the experiences of the two examples given their differing settings and contexts. Think about a health advocacy issue relevant to your area and reflect on how the enabling factors and barriers you have identified from your reading relate to this issue.

Feedback

You may discover that the advocacy faltered or was not as effective as desired owing to a lack of dedicated human resources or the power and money available in the opposing camp. Or, you may find that a passionate, charismatic champion single-handedly was able to galvanize people to act on an issue. You may discover that an unforeseen event, such as an election, had an impact on the advocacy and its outcomes. And you may find that the advocacy managed to use the enabling factors to deal with the potential barriers.

Summary

Our world is becoming more and more complex. The issues that affect human health require more sophisticated and innovative approaches. Health advocacy has been and remains a key factor in successful health promotion interventions. Advocacy needs to build on lessons generated by analysis of what has worked and not worked in the past. In addition, more attention needs to be paid to how we can measure the impact of advocacy action on health. Public health professionals and others also need to acknowledge that advocacy for health issues forms part of our professional roles and responsibilities. After all, if we do not advocate for improved public health outcomes, who will?

References

Alberta Health Services (2009) *Public Health Advocacy*. Health Public Policy Discussion Paper [http://www.albertahealthservices.ca/poph/hi-poph-hpp-public-health-advocacy.pdf; accessed 4 September 2014].

Avery, B. and Bashir, S. (2003) The road to advocacy – searching for the rainbow, *American Journal of Public Health*, 93 (8): 1207–10.

Bassett, M.T. (2003) Public health advocacy, *American Journal of Public Health*, 93 (8): 1204.

Cameron, D. and Jones, I.G. (1983) John Snow, the Broad Street pump and modern epidemiology, *International Journal of Epidemiology*, 12 (3): 393–6.

Canadian Public Health Association (CPHA) (2010) *Leadership in Public Health: A Guide to Advocacy for Public Health Associations*. Ottawa: CPHA [www.cpha.ca/uploads/progs/_/sopha/advocacy-booklet-colour-en-final.pdf; accessed 4 September 2014].

Canadian Public Health Association (CPHA) (2011) *The Public Health Association Movement: 25 Years of Building a Civil Society Voice for Public Health*. Ottawa: CPHA [www.cpha.ca/uploads/progs/_/sopha/sopha_publication_s.pdf; accessed 4 September 2014].

Carlisle, S. (2000) Health promotion, advocacy and health inequalities: a conceptual framework, *Health Promotion International*, 15 (4): 369–76.

Chapman, S. (2001) Advocacy in public health: roles and challenges, *International Journal of Epidemiology*, 30 (6): 1226–32.

Chapman, S. (2004) Advocacy for public health: a primer, *Journal of Epidemiology and Community Health*, 58: 361–5.

Conley-Wright, A. and Jaffe, K.J. (2014) *Six Steps to Successful Child Advocacy: Changing the World for Children*. London: Sage.

Conley-Wright, A. and Taylor, S. (2014) Advocacy by parents of young children with special needs: activities, processes and perceived effectiveness, *Journal of Social Science Research*, 40 (5): 591–605.

Connecticut Association of Nonprofits (CANP) (2003) *Advocacy vs. Lobbying, Coalition Building and Public Engagement*. Hartford, CT: CANP [www.ctnonprofits.org/ctnonprofits/sites/default/files/fckeditor/file/policy/resources/AdvocacyVsLobbying.pdf; accessed 4 September 2014].

Department of Agriculture, Fisheries and Forestry (DAFF) (2013) *National Food Plan: Our Food Future*. Canberra, ACT: DAFF [http://www.daff.gov.au/__data/assets/pdf_file/0011/2293328/national-food-plan-white-paper.pdf; accessed 4 September 2014].

Food & Water Watch (2014) *Global Frackdown Event Planning Guide* [http://www.globalfrackdown.org; accessed 4 September 2014].

Independent Sector (2012) *Beyond the Cause: The Art and Science of Advocacy*. Washington, DC: Independent Sector [https://www.independentsector.org/beyond_the_cause; accessed 4 September 2014].

Minister of Justice (2006) *Lobbying Act 1985*, Chapter 44, s. 5 (4th suppl.). Ottawa: Government of Canada [http://laws.justice.gc.ca/PDF/L-12.4.pdf; accessed 4 September 2014].

Moore, M., Yeatman, H. and Pollard, C. (2013) Evaluating success in public health advocacy strategies, *Vietnam Journal of Public Health*, 1 (1): 66–75.

Moore, S. (2011) Can public-policy advocacy be taught? Or learned?, *The Philanthropist*, 23 (4): 471–80.

Moore, S. (undated) *Improving the Non-Profit, Voluntary and Charitable Sector's Effectiveness in Influencing Decisions of Government*. Edmonton: The Muttart Foundation [www.advocacyschool.org/PDF/MuttartPaperAdvocacy.pdf; accessed 4 September 2014].

National Health and Medical Research Council (NHMRC) (2013) *Australian Dietary Guidelines*. Canberra, ACT: NHMRC [https://www.nhmrc.gov.au/guidelines/publications/n55; accessed 4 September 2014].

Program for Appropriate Technology for Health (PATH) (2013) *Policy Advocacy for Health: A workshop curriculum on policy advocacy strategy development: (1) Facilitator's Guide, (2) Participant's Workbook, (3) Training of Facilitators Manual*. Washington, DC: PATH [www.path.org/publications/detail.php?i=2274; accessed 4 September 2014].

Public Health Agency of Canada (PHAC) (undated) *Public Health Practice: Glossary of Terms*. Ottawa: Government of Canada [www.phac-aspc.gc.ca/php-psp/ccph-cesp/glos-eng.php#a; accessed 4 September 2014].

Public Health Association of Australia (PHAA) (2009) *A Future for Food: Addressing Public Health, Sustainability and Equity from Paddock to Plate* [http://www.phaa.net.au/documents/PHAA%20Report.pdf; accessed 4 September 2014].

Public Health Association of Australia (PHAA) (2011) *Submission of the Public Health Association of Australia on the Tobacco Plain Packaging Bill 2011* [http://www.phaa.net.au/documents/TobaccoPlainpackagingsubHoR.pdf].

Public Health Association of Australia (PHAA) (2012) *A Future for Food 2: Healthy. Sustainable. Fair* [http://www.phaa.net.au/documents/120214%20PHAA%20Report%202012_low%20res.pdf; accessed 4 September 2014].

Sekimpi, D.K., Nkonge, D. and Caceres, L. (2012) *Developing workplace and health facility smoke-free policy environments in Uganda*. Presentation to the 2012 CPHA Annual Conference, Edmonton, 14 June [http://resources.cpha.ca/CPHA/Conf/Data/2012/A12-597e.pdf; accessed 4 September 2014].

Senkubuge, F., Ayo-Yusuf, O.A. and Louwagie, G. (2012) *Smoke free health establishments and determinants of tobacco use among medical students in South Africa*. Presentation to the 13th World Congress on Public Health, Addis Ababa, 27 April [https://wfpha.confex.com/wfpha/2012/webprogram/Paper10769.html; accessed 4 September 2014].

Shepherd, B. (2013) Advocacy: the dark art of influencing policy, *The Guardian*, 28 June [http://www.theguardian.com/global-development-professionals-network/2013/jun/28/advocacy-how-to-influence-government-policy; accessed 4 September 2014].

Stone, D. (1989) Causal stories and the formation of policy agendas, *Political Science Quarterly*, 104 (2): 281–300.

Treatment Action Campaign (TAC) (2003–2014) *Annual Reports*. London: TAC [http://www.tac.org.za/community/annualreports].

United States Senate (1995) *Lobbying Disclosure Act of 1995*, Section 3 Lobbying Definitions [2 U.S.C. 1602]. Washington, DC: United States Senate [www.senate.gov/legislative/Lobbying/Lobby_Disclosure_Act/compilation.pdf; accessed 4 September 2014].

Wallack, L., Dorfman, L., Jernigan, D. and Themba-Nixon, M. (1993) *Media Advocacy and Public Health: Power for Prevention*. London: Sage.

Webster, J., Dunford, E., Kennington, S., Neal, B. and Chapman, S. (2014) Drop the salt! Assessing the impact of a public health advocacy strategy on an Australian government policy on salt, *Public Health Nutrition*, 17(1): 212–18.

World Federation of Public Health Associations (WFPHA) (2011) *Survey of Member Public Health Associations Concerning Policy Advocacy* (unpublished).

World Health Organization (WHO) (1986) *Ottawa Charter for Health Promotion*. Geneva: WHO [http://www.who.int/healthpromotion/conferences/previous/ottawa/en/; accessed 4 September 2014].

World Health Organization (WHO) (1995) *Advocacy Strategies for Health and Development: Development Communication in Action*. Geneva: WHO.

Further reading

Chauvin, J., Hilson, M. and Rosene, C. (2005) Developing civil society's voice for public health, in S.G. Scintee and A. Galan (eds.) *Public Health Strategies: A Tool for Regional Development*. Lage, Germany: Hans Jacobs Verlag.

Christer, H. and Bosse, P. (2011) Public health associations can make a difference: a tribute to the Canadian contributions and some future challenges for public health associations (Commentary), *Journal of Public Health Policy*, 32 (3): 380–90.

Christoffel, K.K. (2000) Public health advocacy: process and product, *American Journal of Public Health*, 90 (5): 722–6.

Public Health Agency of Canada (PHAC) (undated) *Public Health Practice: Glossary of Terms*. Ottawa: Government of Canada [www.phac-aspc.gc.ca/php-psp/ccph-cesp/glos-eng.php#a; accessed 4 September 2014].

Technical Assistance for Civil Society Organisations (TACSO) (2010) *Advocacy and Lobbying*. Sarajevo, BiH: TACSO [www.tacso.org/knowhow/advocacy-lobbing/default.aspx?id=27&template_id=73&langTag=en-US&pageIndex=1].

Toronto Department of Public Health (TDPH) (1991) *Advocacy for Basic Health Prerequisites*. Policy paper. Toronto: TDPH. Cited in McCubbin, M., Labonte, R. and Dallaire, B. (2001) Advocacy for Healthy Public Policy as a Health Promotion Technology. Toronto: University of Toronto Centre for Health Promotion [www.utoronto.ca/chp/symposium.htm].

World Federation of Public Health Associations (WFPHA) (2012) *Annual Report 2011: Public Health Associations – Making the Difference*. Geneva: WFPHA [www.wfpha.org/tl_files/doc/about/wfpha_2011_annual_report_A4_final-3.pdf].

7 Healthy settings

Elaine Gardner

Overview

This chapter explains the concept of healthy settings. This concept focuses on the broad determinants of health-related behaviours at a population level. It has moved from the more traditional view of settings as 'locations' to a broader idea of 'environments' that comprise a number of linked physical spaces. The chapter goes on to discuss some of the advantages and disadvantages of a healthy settings approach. It explains why this is a popular approach to health promotion, reflecting its principal values. The chapter then describes how to go about developing a healthy setting intervention and introduces specific tools that support this process.

Learning objectives

After reading this chapter, you will be able to:

- understand the key principles of the healthy settings approach
- identify examples of settings and environments
- review the advantages and disadvantages of healthy settings approaches
- compare a variety of health-promoting settings and environments
- analyse examples of tools that are useful for development of a settings approach

Key terms

ANGELO framework: Analysis Grid for Elements [previously Environments] Linked to Obesity (Swinburn *et al.*, 1999). A standardized assessment tool for analysing environments and their impact on obesity.

Health equity: The absence of preventable health inequalities.

Obesogenic environment: The role environmental factors can play in determining both nutrition and physical activity.

Settings: Physical environments with an organizational structure where people have defined roles.

Overview of healthy settings

The concept of healthy settings stems from the Ottawa Charter for Health Promotion (WHO, 1986) and was defined as 'The place or social context in which people engage in daily activities in which environmental, organizational and personal factors interact to affect health and wellbeing' (WHO, 1998). The term 'settings' often refers to physical environments with an organizational structure where people have defined roles. The physical environment can be actively influenced and so provide opportunities to solve problems related to health. Actions can be directed at achieving changes in knowledge, attitudes, beliefs, practices, and behaviours of individuals to impact on health behaviour. They can be directed at achieving changes to the physical environment or changes to an organizational structure through, for example, policies, laws, and power structures. Actions can also be directed at achieving a combination of these changes. Settings also offer the opportunity to reach specific target populations such as risk-identified individuals or networks, or those who work, study or socialize in a particular setting.

Recently, online social networking sites (SNS) have been suggested as 'novel settings' that could be used to influence health. They certainly fulfil the WHO definition as a '. . . social context in which people engage in daily activities . . .' (WHO, 1998), and Loss *et al.* (2014) argue that the social interaction facilitated by online SNS may increasingly be more important than physical boundaries when defining a 'setting'. Social networking sites may increase participation in health by allowing people to create their own content, but Loss *et al.* (2014) do caution that exposure to risky behaviours through widespread communication with peers could also cause the SNS environment to be detrimental to health. Other requirements of a settings approach to health, such as building partnerships and changing the environment, have yet to be explored with SNS, as currently its use tends to rely on health education directed at end users.

 Activity 7.1

Consider the definition of a 'setting' and compile a list of examples. Try and include a range of different types of settings.

Feedback

A number of existing World Health Organization (WHO) healthy settings approaches are identified in Figure 7.1. Other settings you may have thought of include night clubs, sports clubs, homes, children's centres, activity centres, and other 'diffuse, virtual settings and contexts where people Google, shop and travel' (Kickbusch, 1997). 'Supportive environments' are also included (as discussed below).

You may have identified other examples of settings. Crucially, a setting is part of the environment around us that may be shaped to improve health. Opportunities exist to change these spaces and social contexts to positively impact on our health.

The principles of the healthy settings approach

The healthy settings approach adopts an ecological approach to health that sees health as the dynamic product of interactions between individuals and their environments (Dooris, 2005). It focuses on interventions at a community or population level to identify goals that focus on changes in organizations, systems, and the environment and therefore on the broader determinants of health, rather than simply addressing individual and population behavioural risk factors. This involves a shift in emphasis from individual health problems and topic-based factors to the nature of the system and organization. The

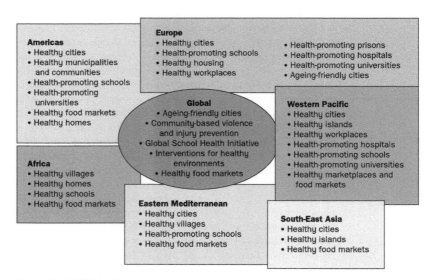

Figure 7.1 WHO healthy settings approaches.

Reproduced from WHO (2014) with the permission of the World Health Organization.

settings approach is underpinned by health promotion values such as empowerment, public participation, equity, and partnership. It places emphasis on developing personal competencies, implementing policies effectively, reshaping environments, building partnerships for sustainable change, and facilitating ownership of change throughout the setting (Whitelaw *et al.*, 2001).

Healthy settings initiatives work towards the improvement of a variety of health risk factors simultaneously, so they have a holistic and multi-disciplinary approach to health improvement. Health risk factors can have a singular or specific focus, but are more likely to encompass a variety of health improvement areas such as physical activity, nutrition, drug awareness, alcohol and tobacco use, pollution, violence (including bullying), sexual health and mental health issues.

Developing supportive environments

A specific setting may have limited capacity to address the wider determinants of health. As a result, a broader approach of 'supportive environments' for health has developed. This recognizes that links and connections exist between settings and that people do not interact in just one setting, so a joined-up approach is crucial. Health issues do not respect organizational or geographical boundaries. By networking horizontally to make links with other settings, effective health promotion is enabled, avoiding duplication of effort and wastage of resources.

Healthy settings should focus on policies and practices that will create supportive environments, alongside public health action at a local level that allows broad community involvement and control. An example of the development of a supportive environment is the programme 'Healthy People, Healthy Places' (Public Health England, 2013), which provides ideas for actions by council bodies and local authorities, to ensure that health, well-being, and inequalities are addressed in the planning and development of the built environment. Figure 7.2 shows another example developed by the Town and Country Planning Association, which draws together the links between public health objectives and potential 'places' interventions to support this development (Ross and Chang, 2013).

The importance of a whole-system approach

An intervention within a particular setting is different from a healthy settings approach. Interventions using the healthy settings approach are holistic in that they consider all the interrelationships, interactions, and interdependencies within a setting as a whole, rather than focusing on these separately. This is because these individual parts can only be fully understood in relation to the whole. This can result in complex interactions that cross organizational boundaries and engage with the wider environment, as Figure 7.2 demonstrates. Within the remit of planners to create health-promoting built environments, there are recommendations involving wide-ranging health areas such as safety, community spirit, food outlets, green spaces, traffic, waste disposal, health care provision, access, lighting, energy efficiency, local industries, allotments for growing food, and noise pollution. All of these topics are important in their own right but change can be maximized if they are examined as a whole. It should be acknowledged, however, that the sheer enormity and diversity of a whole-system approach means that it can be difficult to manage and at times unpredictable. But the rewards of such an approach can be summed up in the phrase attributed to the ancient Greek philosopher Aristotle: 'the whole is greater than the sum of its parts'.

Developing a healthy settings intervention

The tasks involved in planning and delivering any health promotion intervention also apply to one using a healthy settings approach. These are discussed in Section 1 of this book. However, some areas need particular consideration when planning interventions using a healthy settings approach.

Health needs assessment is crucial in planning an intervention using a healthy settings approach. This also needs to incorporate a systematic analysis of environmental influences and organizational capacity. Such a systematic analysis can create opportunities for empowerment and capacity building with those in the settings as well as other stakeholders. Poland et al. (2009) have developed an analytical framework covering three main areas: understanding settings; changing settings; and knowledge development and translation. This framework can be used with people in the setting to promote discussion, as well as being useful as a quick assessment tool for the practitioner. Another analytical tool is the ANGELO framework, which is described in Activity 7.4.

The healthy settings approach requires the involvement of multiple stakeholders throughout the whole process from the initial consultation through to the programme design, goal setting, implementation, monitoring, and evaluation. This presents challenges around coordination and communication and there may also be conceptual differences in how success is defined. For example, in a workplace setting this would include the views of all types and levels of workers (manual, administration, professional, management, catering personnel, cleaning staff), the unions, suppliers, and purchasers. Different groups may measure success differently. For example, absenteeism rates might be a more important indicator of success for management, and choice of food in

Figure 7.2 Ways in which planners can create health-promoting environments.

Category	Reduce obesity, diabetes, and heart and circulatory disease (Table 1)	Promote good mental health and wellbeing (Table 2)	Reduce health inequalities (Table 3)	Improve the health of an ageing population (Table 4)	Reduce the incidence of respiratory diseases (Table 5)	Reduce traffic-related injuries (Table 6)	Improve the provision of, and access to, healthcare facilities (Table 7)
Economically active places Accessible and fulfilling local employment and training opportunities. Town centres that have vitality and viability.	✓✓	✓✓	✓✓	✓✓			
Sociable places Opportunities for people to meet others, socialize and organize together.	✓	✓	✓	✓			✓
Environmentally sustainable places Neighbourhoods with low levels of air and water pollution, noise and contamination. Networks of green and blue infrastructure, including parks, play areas and open spaces, roof gardens, street trees and water features. Neighbourhoods/homes that are adapted to the impacts of a changing climate, such as flooding and excessive heat and cold. Homes that are dry and energy efficient.	✓✓	✓✓✓	✓✓	✓✓	✓✓	✓	
Well designed places A public realm that is attractive and safe. Good-quality homes that can be adapted to people's changing circumstances. Places that are locally distinctive and foster a strong identity of place. Step-free pedestrian routes with benches and public toilets. Well designed healthcare facilities that have views onto/connections to green infrastructure networks.	✓	✓✓✓	✓✓	✓✓	✓✓	✓	✓
Accessible and active places Well connected, active and sustainable travel options to local facilities and services. New, large-scale, mixed-use development based around public transport, cycling and walking. Child-friendly 20 mph urban environments with convenient access to schools and play opportunities. Street patterns and layout in which walking and cycling are the easy, default choices. Convenient access to healthcare, which may include co-locating facilities with other services.	✓✓✓	✓✓✓	✓✓✓	✓✓	✓✓✓	✓✓✓	✓✓
Inclusive places Neighbourhoods of people with the poorest health benefiting most from a targeted approach to improve the local environment. Availability of healthy food and opportunities to grow one's own food. Restrictions on unhealthy uses that are disproportionately located in deprived areas, such as payday lenders, betting shops and hot-food takeaways.	✓✓	✓✓	✓	✓	✓	✓	✓

the canteen might be more important for workers. Stakeholders' involvement is important so that different viewpoints are understood and incorporated. Widening the ownership at all levels and in all aspects of the process of planning the intervention helps build capacity for delivery and achieve sustainability.

Since the healthy settings approach is characterized by a focus on system change and creating more supportive environments, multiple interventions, programmes, and levels will be involved. This means several different planning cycles will be required.

In addition, different strands of the programme will have different measurement priorities for evaluation. To take account of these different priorities, the need to develop a sound evidence base, and an ecological approach based on broad system change, an overarching evaluation framework is needed. This should include input from stakeholders. It also needs key indicators that are valid, meaningful, and credible. These indicators and other evaluation measures need to be appropriate for the setting, its context, and its requirement to examine the processes that deliver change, as well as the synergies that may occur. Outcomes need to be measured at different levels (individual, organizational, policy, and community). Table 7.1 provides an example of a framework for an evaluation.

As already explained, there are a variety of settings that can be used in a healthy setting intervention. Some of the most common settings are now described in more detail.

Schools as healthy settings

The World Health Organization introduced the idea of Health Promoting Schools (HPS) in the early 1980s, and in 1992 the European Health Promoting Schools Network was established. Since that time, other networks throughout the world have adopted the concept of HPS (Deschesnes et al., 2003). The approach is used to educate and influence young people, with the advantage of being able to access them at an early age and continue to work with them over many years. The WHO developed a framework for action (WHO, 2009) and updated the principles of HPS (WHO, 2011). These principles recognize that it is important to do more than offer health education classes in the curriculum if HPS are to be truly successful. Figure 7.3 shows the interaction of the key factors involved in HPS. Rowe et al. (2007: 524) conclude that the HPS approach 'has the potential to build school connectedness through two major mechanisms: inclusive processes that involve the diversity of members that make up a community . . . and supportive structures such as school policies'. Different tools are available for monitoring and assessing progress in HPS, some of which have been reviewed by Young and colleagues, who conclude: 'the tools most likely to be successful and sustainable need to have considered ownership and cultural issues and therefore involved practitioners in the development' (Young et al., 2012: 10).

There are HPS initiatives throughout the world, and regional networks for the development of HPS have been initiated in Europe, the Western Pacific, and Latin America by WHO. A systematic review of the effectiveness of school-based nutrition promotion programmes has shown that HPS can increase the consumption of healthier foods (such as water, milk, fruit, and vegetables) and reduce behaviours such as 'breakfast skipping', intake of low-nutrient, energy-dense foods, and eating disorders (Wang and Stewart, 2013). In Zhejiang Province, China, Wang et al. (2013) found that although using a health education approach in isolation can increase nutrition knowledge among middle-school students, parents, and staff, HPS was more effective and had a positive impact on students' eating behaviours, in addition to their knowledge.

Table 7.1 A processing framework for evaluation of Healthy Cities projects (Department of Health, 2010)

Structures: Set-up	Process: Activities	Output: Short-term achievements	Outcome: Long-term achievements
Organizational capacity (project office; accountable mechanism) Stable resources: (funding; inter-sectoral parnerships; community ownership)	Identify health needs and target group Plan project strategy Encourage community participation Promote innovation Evaluate project effectiveness Share experiences	Activity completed as planned Review project objectives Compare knowledge, attitude, and practice change before and after activity	Underscore the specific individual, communal or environmental health outcomes that are likely to take a longer time to achieve
Examples of indicators	*Examples of indicators*	*Examples of indicators*	*Examples of indicators*
Set up project office Build a representative steering committee Secure project funding	Make a community diagnosis Activities implemented (number of seminars, workshops) Number of target recipients receiving the intervention	Increased number of schools setting up a policy on healthy eating Increased level of physical activity of participants Increased consumption of fruit and vegetables by participants	Decline in mortality and morbidity rates of communicable and non-communicable diseases Improved air quality as demonstrated by decline in air pollution index Decreased overweight and obesity rates

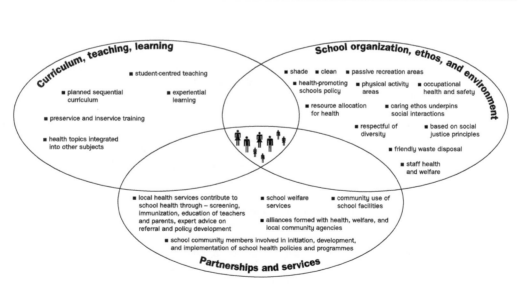

Figure 7.3 Framework to demonstrate the contribution of whole-school approaches embodied by the health-promoting school approach.

Reproduced from Rowe, F., Stewart, D., Patterson, C. (2007) Promoting school contentedness through whole school approaches with the permission of Emerald Group Publishing Limited.

Workplaces as healthy settings

Interventions using a healthy settings approach can be effective in the workplace. Although they exclude specific age groups, such as children and adults past retirement age, and are limited to those employed in workplaces participating in workplace health setting initiatives, they do have the potential to reach large parts of the adult population from different social backgrounds. It must also be noted that adults spend a considerable amount of time at work.

The implementation of workplace health promotion provides health benefits and potential reductions in absenteeism, which can result in increased productivity and reduced costs for the employer, so it makes good business sense. However, it does require a commitment by employers to address the organizational sources of worker ill health, for example long-hours or bullying, so that health becomes an integral part of the organization. A validated tool for workplace health needs assessment, which can be amended for use in different organizations and includes a useful framework for creating a healthy workplace, has been developed by the Department of Health in England (DoH, 2012).

✎ Activity 7.2

The abstract below and Figure 7.4 are taken from an article about healthy workplaces in northern India (Thakur et al., 2012: 108). Read the abstract and reflect on how effective you think it is as a healthy settings approach in the workplace.

'**Background:** Keeping in view of rapid industrialization and growing Indian economy, there has been a substantial increase in the workforce in India. Currently there is no organized workplace model for promoting health of industrial workers in India. **Objective:** To develop and implement a healthy workplace model in three industrial settings of North India. **Materials and Methods:** An operations research was conducted for 12 months in purposively selected three industries of Chandigarh. In phase I, a multi-stakeholder workshop was conducted to finalize the components and tools for the healthy workplace model. NCD [non-communicable disease] risk factors were assessed in 947 employees in these three industries. In phase II, the healthy workplace model was implemented on pilot basis for a period of 12 months in these three industries to finalize the model. **Findings:** Healthy workplace committee with involvement of representatives of management, labor union and research organization was formed in three industries. Various tools like comprehensive and rapid healthy workplace assessment forms, NCD work-lite format for risk factors surveillance and monitoring and evaluation format were developed. The prevalence of tobacco use [and] alcoholics was found to be 17.8% and 47%, respectively. Around one-third (28%) of employees complained of back pain in the past 12 months. Healthy workplace model with focus on three key components (physical environment, psychosocial work environment, and promoting healthy habits) was developed, implemented on pilot basis, and finalized based on experience in participating industries. A stepwise approach for model with a core, expanded, and optional components were also suggested. An accreditation system is also required for promoting healthy workplace program. **Conclusion:** Integrated healthy workplace model is feasible, could be implemented in industrial setting in northern India and needs to be pilot tested in other parts of the country.'

Feedback

Using the industrial workplace as a setting meant that a large and increasing population was targeted that may not have been accessed via other sources. The results show a high level of health needs with regards to addiction and physical pain. Other areas, such as mental stress and absenteeism, are not cited in the abstract. There is commitment by management to the programme, as demonstrated initially by their participation in the study, then by changes in their practices, by adapting the structures of their committees to include employees and by the development of different tools. A healthy workplace model was developed that focused on three key components: the physical environment; the psychosocial work environment; and promoting healthy habits. Although the abstract does not provide more detail about these environments, Figure 7.4 indicates that their spread is extensive, interlinked, and addresses a range of the determinants of health. The programme is indeed a whole-system approach.

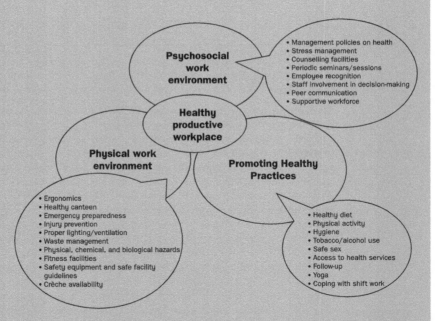

Figure 7.4 Model for healthy workplace in an industrial setting in northern India.

Reproduced from Thakur *et al.* (2012) with the permission of the *Indian Journal of Occupational and Environmental Medicine.*

Neighbourhoods as healthy settings

Neighbourhoods or communities are more fluid and less defined entities than settings such as cities but they can still be used in a healthy settings approach. Although they may be enclosed by geographical boundaries, these are often defined by agencies external to a community, for example boundaries used for administrative and election purposes. A community tends to have a common bond and is defined by its collective needs and priorities and its shared responsibilities in tackling these.

A healthy setting approach based on a community is slightly different from a community development approach because it requires a location to bring people together, which may be a neighbourhood. Neighbourhoods offer an infrastructure for health, opportunities to access vulnerable groups such as older people or those on a low income, a potential for priorities to be set by residents rather than professionals, and opportunities to tackle the social determinants of health. These social determinants of health are discussed in more detail in Chapter 5. An example of a healthy neighbourhood scheme is the Communities for Health Programme in England (IDeA, 2009), where disadvantaged communities are involved in adopting healthier lifestyles and are empowered to take more responsibility for improving their own health.

A healthy settings approach is different from interventions delivered within a community or neighbourhood, as it uses the whole-system approach described earlier in this chapter to address the interrelated environments. For example, a healthy settings approach in a neighbourhood that seeks to develop healthy eating at a local level may look at the social norms that influence food choice, fewer fast-food restaurants being permitted to open, the nutritional labelling of menus, the allocation of space and facilities for a regular fruit and vegetable market, and subsidies in local shops for the purchase of healthy food items.

✎ Activity 7.3

'Obesity and the Environment Briefing: Regulating the Growth of Fast Food Outlets' (Public Health England, 2013) suggests that there are three broad approaches that could be taken to address the problem of the increasing numbers of hot-food takeaways in city centres and near schools:

- working with the takeaway businesses and food industry to make food healthier;
- working with schools to reduce fast food consumed by children; and
- using regulatory and planning measures to address the proliferation of hot food takeaways.

Answer the following questions:

(1) Suggest reasons why hot-food takeaways may have a detrimental impact on health.
(2) Consider the three approaches suggested, and describe what in your opinion is the best approach to reduce the problem.

Feedback

(1) There are a number of reasons you might have suggested why hot-food takeaways may have a detrimental impact on health, including those noted in the paper (Public Health England, 2013) and other research on this issue (Fraser et al., 2010). These include:

- Generate substantial litter in a neighbourhood;
- Discarded food waste and litter attracts foraging animals and pests;
- Reduce the visual appeal of the local environment;
- Generate night-time noise;
- Generate unacceptable levels of cooking smells;
- Contribute to traffic congestion and accidents due to short-term parking outside takeaways;
- Contribute to health inequalities in deprived communities, as there is a strong association between deprivation and the density of fast food outlets.

Additionally, it should be noted that hot-food takeaways often serve energy-dense food and there has been an increase in the proportion of high-calorie food consumed outside the home. This contributes to the increasing prevalence of obesity and non-communicable disease (NCDs). The local food environment around children's homes has an independent effect on child weight status (Miller *et al.*, 2014).

(2) Working with takeaway businesses and the food industry to make food healthier can have an impact on healthier food consumption, but it is a slow process, the potential for change is limited, and there tends to be varying levels of success. The UK Responsibility Deal is an example of a voluntary agreement between businesses and government to increase the availability of healthier food (DoH, 2011). Many business owners are unwilling or unable to make major changes owing to increased costs, perceived consumer demand, and adverse effects on profitability.

Working with schools to encourage pupils through education to reduce their fast food intake has been tried worldwide with varying degrees of success. The food industry targets children and their families with heavy marketing and food promotions that can have a counter-effect. In families, knowledge and skills around budgeting, shopping, and preparation of healthy food can also be lacking, so hot food takeaways often replace food prepared at home to feed the family.

Using regulatory and planning measures can have an effect on limiting the number of hot-food takeaways, especially within a certain radius of schools. However, this does not impact on other factors contributing to obesity levels, such as the sale of sweets and fizzy drinks or sedentary behaviour.

Overall, no single approach on its own can achieve the beneficial long-term health outcome of a reduction in obesity levels, although shorter-term health impacts may be improved and there may be an impact on other individual public health issues such as litter, noise, and pest control. Interventions need to link and work together at all levels to improve health and health inequalities.

Cities as healthy settings

In 1987, the World Health Organization launched the Healthy Cities initiative in Europe. Healthy Cities has rapidly grown to become a global movement with over 2000 cities involved. It has been used to design and implement actions that improve and sustain the health and equity of people living and working in urban settings. The Healthy Cities approach is based on the concept that local governments are ideally placed to pursue strategies using holistic ideas of health because their functions closely connect them to the lives of their communities. In addition, they can require all policy areas to show how they contribute to and impact upon population health, including transport, housing, health services, infrastructure, and cultural development.

The Healthy Cities approach recognizes that cities need to be planned, governed, and organized if health is to be high on the political, social, and economic agendas. A Healthy City is defined by how it undertakes these processes rather than outcomes. It does not depend on a city's current health infrastructure, but upon its commitment to improve the city environment. Box 7.1 provides an example of a Healthy City. Evaluation of the Healthy Cities projects has been variable.

Box 7.1 Bogota, Colombia as a Healthy City

In Bogota, the city is being actively transformed in an attempt to promote more physical activity by reducing car dependency and increasing public transport, cycling, and walking. Initiatives include: traffic-free streets, where roads are closed to traffic for fixed periods on Sundays and holidays to increase cycling and walking (this applies to 97 km of its streets); improvements to the public transport systems through the Bus Rapid Transit system, which has both reduced car use and commuter times and also encouraged users to walk longer distances than previously to fixed bus stations; physical improvements in pavements and an increase in green public spaces; and a 334 km cycle path network. These were made possible by a commitment from numerous city administrations to change the built environment and raise the appropriate finance. Unfortunately, the improvements have not been able to keep up with the growth of the population or the number of private vehicles, and still only 44.7% of the population are meeting guidelines for physical activity. Only 2% of daily journeys are made by bicycle, with fear of crime, lack of secure parking facilities, and a perceived high number of traffic deaths among cyclists cited as reasons.

Source: Adapted from Rydin *et al.* (2012)

Many issues that impact on Healthy Cities are driven by forces outside of the city or country and are a result of changes affecting cities globally. Increasing urbanization means more people living in cities than rural areas. Urbanized populations are also living longer, which places increasing demands on health care and long-term care in areas such as housing. Cities are vulnerable to the impacts of changing environmental conditions, including flooding and urban heat island generation, an increase in transportation of both people and freight, which causes a range of problems including air and noise pollution, increased waste disposal and increased accidents. In addition to these global changes that are driven by forces outside of the city or country, city-level decision-making may be weak or inadequate for some necessary leverage change.

There is no single answer to all of these interconnected challenges, as each city is unique in terms of its socio-political dynamics, governance arrangements, priorities, and its ability to mobilize community support. Social inequalities and health inequalities within cities are widening. Health equity, which pays attention to the needs of the vulnerable and socially disadvantaged by addressing preventable health inequalities, is one of the key principles and priorities of Healthy Cities. Numerous examples of interventions to address inequalities in health in cities exist, including free fruit and breakfast for children, improving access to buildings and public transport for the elderly and disabled, race equity schemes, safer routes to school, developing infrastructure to attract new enterprises and jobs, providing new water pipes to ensure high-quality drinking water, free health care check-ups and preventative services for disadvantaged groups, crime reduction programmes, and neighbourhood councils to improve participation in decision-making. Ritsatakis (2009), however, found that there is unfulfilled potential for addressing health inequalities in urban populations, and an urgent need to address longer-term risks to health such as climate change.

Developing a healthy environment: focusing on obesity

The ANGELO framework is an assessment tool for environmental determinants of obesity that can help in the planning process when developing programmes to tackle the obesogenic environment. The framework examines both the micro and macro environment: the 'micro' environment refers to small environments that can be influenced by individuals or small organizations; and the 'macro' environment is the much larger, often industry- or government-level environments. Four types of environments that potentially contribute to obesity are included (physical, economic, policy, and socio-cultural).

Table 7.2 Example of the ANGELO framework: the Pacific Islands

	Physical	*Economic*	*Political*	*Socio-cultural*
Micro environmental				
Festivities				Cultural importance of high-fat foods
Neighbourhoods	Recreation and sports facilities; safe walking paths			
Schools	Canteens serving local foods		Policies on physical education; promotion of traditional activities (e.g. dancing)	
Homes	Home gardens			
Churches				Church leaders as role models
Markets	Availability of local food			
Macro environmental				
Transport system	Availability of buses			
Health Policy			Policies and standards on imported food quality/labelling	

Source: Swinburn *et al.* (1999)

Table 7.3 Example of the ANGELO framework: the United Kingdom

	Physical	Economic	Political	Socio-cultural
Micro environmental				
Family	Availability of 'healthy foods'			Parental eating habits
Neighbourhoods	Recreation and sports facilities; number of fast food outlets		Sports clubs	
Schools	Quality of food served in canteen		Physical education; sports clubs	
Macro environmental				
Industry	Large portion sizes; nutritional content of processed foods			
Media		Food advertising, especially 'unhealthy' foods		
Government		Food taxes; food standards		

Source: Swinburn et al. (1999)

Tables 7.2 and 7.3 provide examples of the ANGELO framework, highlighting priority areas for two different parts of the world: the Pacific Islands and the United Kingdom (Swinburn et al., 1999).

🖉 **Activity 7.4**

Consider the examples of the ANGELO framework shown in Tables 7.2 and 7.3, and refer back to the principles of the healthy settings approach. Does the ANGELO framework support this approach?

Feedback

Consider the original definition of a healthy setting: 'The place or social context in which people engage in daily activities in which environmental, organizational and personal factors interact to affect health and wellbeing' (WHO, 1998). In the examples provided, the framework examines populations rather than individuals, and is related to obesogenic environments commonly found in communities. The focus is on different sizes of organizations, various systems, the environment, and on the broader determinants of health. A holistic approach to prioritizing health improvement is facilitated by the inclusion of four types of interlinked environments. This is demonstrated by the range of coverage in the Pacific Islands, which encompasses such diverse factors as social structures within the church, the infrastructure of transportation, and food availability to government policies on food taxes. By having a logical structure, the interrelationships, interactions, and interdependencies between organizations implicated can be easier to identify and visualize. Within the UK, a different analysis is achieved as would be expected given the difference in context, but it still encompasses the principles outlined. A whole-settings approach is shown.

The ANGELO framework is a tool to analyse and identify priority elements for planning and implementation of a programme, and so is only part of the healthy settings approach to health promotion. It can, however, also contribute to capacity-building and formative evaluation. A representation of how the framework fits into the overall process is shown in Figure 7.5 (Simmons et al., 2009).

Advantages of a healthy settings approach

A settings approach has the following advantages:

- It recognizes that health is influenced by contextual and environmental factors and therefore addresses the range of physical, social, organizational, and cultural factors that impact on health in an environment.
- It offers a positive and participatory approach to health, engaging different stakeholders in the task of making better environments and organizations.
- It embeds health in already established structures and environments with clearly identified locations and boundaries and, as a result, planning may be easier.
- Defined organizational structures will be in place, with groups and networks able to highlight local issues.
- These established networks provide mutual support and so peer education can have a potentially significant impact.
- Some resources may already be defined and in place through the organizational structures, and additional targeted funding may be easier to obtain due to the established nature of the setting.

Limitations of a healthy settings approach

A settings approach has the following limitations:

- It is important to consider that groups within settings may be considered homogenous when in fact they are not. For example, consider the different types of workers in a workplace setting – manual, secretarial, shift workers, young and old – and their levels of physical activity and it will be clear that their health needs are different.
- Marginalized groups such as sex workers, the homeless, the unemployed, and elderly housebound do not access commonly used settings. As a result, using a settings approach could exacerbate health inequalities, particularly among marginalized groups, as they are unlikely to be present in the setting where the intervention takes place.

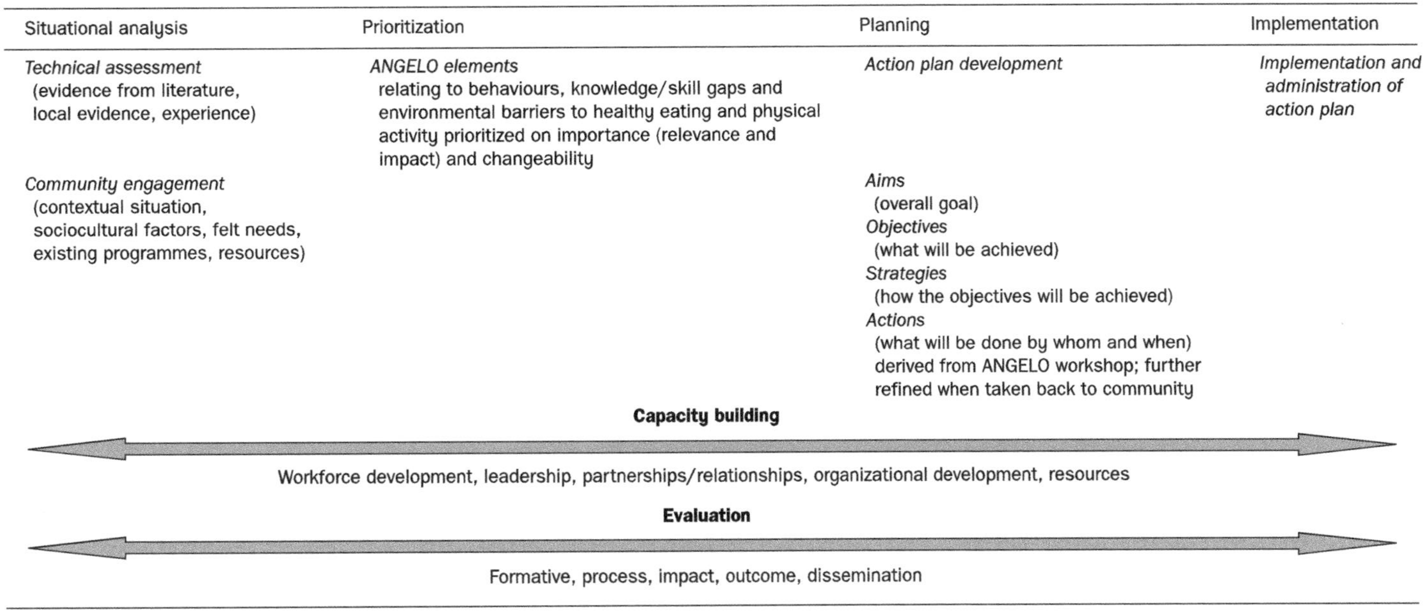

Situational analysis
Prioritization
Planning
Implementation
Technical assessment
(evidence from literature, local evidence, experience)
ANGELO elements
relating to behaviours, knowledge/skill gaps and environmental barriers to healthy eating and physical activity prioritized on importance (relevance and impact) and changeability
Action plan development
Implementation and administration of action plan
Community engagement
(contextual situation, sociocultural factors, felt needs, existing programmes, resources)
Aims
(overall goal)
Objectives
(what will be achieved)
Strategies
(how the objectives will be achieved)
Actions
(what will be done by whom and when) derived from ANGELO workshop; further refined when taken back to community
Capacity building
Workforce development, leadership, partnerships/relationships, organizational development, resources
Evaluation
Formative, process, impact, outcome, dissemination

Figure 7.5 The overall health promotion process highlighting the role of the ANGELO framework.

Reproduced from Simmons *et al.* (2009) with the permission of *Health Promotion International*.

- There may be restrictions to multi-agency and partnership working in particular settings, such as working with certain food companies within a school setting.
- It is challenging to evaluate because it does not fit easily into an epidemiological framework of 'evidence' but needs to be analysed in terms of social and political processes.
- It requires the commitment and active participation of all the stakeholders involved in a setting to be effective.

Summary

The healthy settings approach to health promotion has evolved to incorporate 'environments' and a 'whole-system' approach. The development of an intervention using a healthy settings approach follows the same stages as those associated with other health promotion interventions but can present additional challenges owing to its size, diversity, and multiple stakeholders. Cities, neighbourhoods, and settings such as schools and workplaces can impact on health and have been used in healthy settings initiatives. A change in organizational ethos is essential for interventions to be effective. A healthy settings approach is broad, but a variety of tools exist that can contribute to its development in particular settings and environments.

References

Department of Health (2010) *Evaluating a Healthy Cities Project*. Hong Kong: Government of the Hong Kong Special Administrative Region [www.chp.gov.uk; accessed 11 September 2014].

Department of Health (DoH) (2011) *The Public Health Responsibility Deal*. London: DoH [https://responsibility deal.dh.gov.uk/; accessed 11 September 2014].

Department of Health (DoH) ((2012) *Health Work and Wellbeing – Defining the Priorities: Workplace Health Needs Assessment for Employers*. London: DoH [http://www.regionalplatform.org.uk/write/273_181 Workplace_HNA_for_Employers.pdf; accessed 11 September 2014].

Deschesnes, M., Martin, C. and Jomphe Hill, A. (2003) Comprehensive approaches to school health promotion: how to achieve broader implementation?, *Health Promotion International*, 18 (4): 387–96.

Dooris, M. (2005) Healthy settings: challenges to generating evidence of effectiveness, *Health Promotion International*, 21 (1): 55–64.

Fraser, L., Edwards, K., Cade, J. and Clarke, G. (2010) The geography of fast food outlets: a review, *International Journal of Environmental Research and Public Health*, 7 (5): 2290–308.

Improvement and Development Agency (IDeA) (2009) *Communities for Health: The Story So Far. . ..* London: IDeA.

Kickbusch, I. (1997) Health-promoting environments: the next steps, *Australia and New Zealand Journal of Public Health*, 21: 431–4.

Loss, J., Lindacher, V. and Curbach, J. (2014) Online social networking sites – a novel setting for health promotion?, *Health and Place*, 26: 161–70.

Miller, L., Joyce, S., Carter, S. and Yun, G. (2014) Associations between childhood obesity and the availability of food outlets in the local environment: a retrospective cross-sectional study, *American Journal of Health Promotion*, 28 (6): e137–45.

Poland, B., Krupa, G. and McCall, D. (2009) Settings for health promotion: an analytic framework to guide intervention design and implementation, *Health Promotion Practice*, 10: 505–16.

Public Health England (PHE) (2013) *Obesity and the Environment Briefing: Regulating the Growth of Fast Food Outlets*. London: PHE [https://www.gov.uk/government/publications/obesity-and-the-environment-briefing-regulating-the-growth-of-fast-food-outlets; accessed 11 September 2014].

Ritsatakis, A. (2009) Equity and social determinants of health at city level, *Health Promotion International*, 24 (suppl. 1): i81–90.

Ross, A. and Chang, M. (2013) *Planning Healthier Places*. London: Town and Country Planning Association [http://www.tcpa.org.uk/data/files/Health_and_planning/Health_Phase_2/Planning_Healthier_Places .pdf; accessed 11 September 2014].

Rowe, F., Stewart, D. and Patterson, C. (2007) Promoting school connectedness through whole school approaches, *Health Education*, 107 (6): 524–42.

Rydin, Y., Bleahu, A., Davies, M., Dávila, J.D., Friel, S., De Grandis, G. *et al.* (2012) Shaping cities for health: complexity and the planning of urban environments in the 21st century, *The Lancet*, 379 (9831): 2079–2108.

Simmons, A., Mavoa, H.M. and Bell, A.C. (2009) Creating community action plans for obesity prevention using the ANGELO (Analysis Grid for Elements Linked to Obesity) Framework, *Health Promotion International*, 24 (4): 311–24.

Swinburn, B., Egger, G. and Raza, F. (1999) Dissecting obesogenic environments: the development and application of a framework for identifying and prioritising environmental interventions for obesity, *Preventative Medicine*, 29: 563–70.

Thakur, J.S., Bains, P., Kar, S.S., Wadhwa, S., Moirangthem, P., Kumar, R. *et al.* (2012) Integrated healthy workplace model: an experience from North Indian industry, *Indian Journal of Occupational and Environmental Medicine*, 16 (3): 108–13.

Wang, D. and Stewart, D. (2013) The implementation and effectiveness of school-based nutrition promotion programmes using a health-promoting school approach: a systematic review, *Public Health Nutrition*, 16 (6): 1082–100.

Wang, D., Stewart, D., Yuan, Y. and Chang, C. (2013) Do health promoting schools improve nutrition in China?, *Health Promotion International* (DOI:10.1093/heapro/dat047).

Whitelaw, S., Baxendale, A., Bryce, C., MacHardy, L., Young, I. and Witney, E. (2001) 'Settings' based health promotion: a review, *Health Promotion International*, 16 (4): 339–53.

World Health Organization (WHO) (1986) *Ottawa Charter for Health Promotion*. Geneva: WHO [http://www.who. int/healthpromotion/conferences/previous/ottawa/en/].

World Health Organization (WHO) (1998) *Health Promotion Glossary*. Geneva: WHO [http://www.who.int/ healthpromotion/about/HPG/en/; accessed 11 September 2014].

World Health Organization (WHO) (2009) *Health Promoting Schools: A Framework for Action* [http://www.wpro. who.int/health_promotion/about/health_promoting_schools_framework/en/; accessed 11 September 2014].

World Health Organization (WHO) (2011) *What is a Health Promoting School?* Geneva: WHO [http://www.who. int/school_youth_health/gshi/hps/en/index.html; accessed 11 September 2014].

World Health Organization (WHO) (2014) *Regional Activities: Approaches as Implemented in the WHO Regions*. Geneva: WHO [http://www.who.int/healthy_settings/regional/en/; accessed 11 September 2014].

Young, I., St. Leger, L. and Blanchard, C. (2012) *Monitoring and Assessing Progress in Health Promoting Schools: Issues for Policy-makers to Consider*. Saint Denis, France: IUHPE [http://www.iuhpe.org/index.php/en/ iuhpe-thematic-resources/298-on-school-health; accessed 11 September 2014].

8 Developing healthy communities through community mobilization

Morten Skovdal and Paula Valentine

Overview

The aim of this chapter is to address the role of community mobilization in developing healthy communities. The chapter provides a brief overview of community mobilization before moving on to introduce various tools and methods that can be used to mobilize communities. The chapter then illustrates how these tools can be applied in practice through a discussion of 'real world' projects. The chapter ends with a discussion of some of the challenges involved.

Learning objectives

After reading this chapter, you will be able to:

- explain the characteristics of community mobilization and its role in building healthy communities
- plan a programme that builds healthy communities through community mobilization
- understand how to use a variety of participatory tools to mobilize a community for better health
- describe the strengths and challenges inherent to community mobilization

Key terms

Community: A group of people who have something in common, such as living in the same geographical area or sharing common attitudes, interests or lifestyles.

Community development: An approach to development that seeks to increase the extent and effectiveness of community action, community activity, and agencies' relationships with communities.

Community mobilization: A capacity-building process through which local individuals, groups or organizations identify needs, plan, carry out and evaluate activities on a participatory and sustained basis, so as to improve health and other needs, based on their own initiative or stimulated by others.

Community participation: A process (and approach) whereby community members assume a level of responsibility and become agents for their own health and development.

> **Participatory Learning and Action (PLA):**   A collection of methods and approaches used in action research, which enable diverse groups and individuals to learn, work, and act together in a cooperative manner, to focus on issues of joint concern, identify challenges, and generate positive responses in a collaborative and democratic manner.

Characteristics of community mobilization

Early health promotion efforts were guided by strategies focused on individual-level behaviour change. However, as Chapter 5 explained, the Alma Ata Declaration of 1978 introduced a shift in thinking, recognizing the role of socio-economic and cultural factors in determining the health behaviour and practices of individuals, groups, and communities (WHO, 1978). This shift was further supported by the 1986 Ottawa Charter (WHO, 1986) and the 2005 Bangkok Charter (WHO, 2005). These Charters cemented a participatory rhetoric in public health, giving rise to community mobilization in health promotion. The theoretical underpinning of community mobilization as a means of health promotion is described in chapter 6 of *Health Promotion Theory* in the Understanding Public Health series (Skovdal, 2013).

Community mobilization means different things to different people and programmes therefore take different forms. Campbell (2014) highlights four approaches to community mobilization:

- *Instrumental approaches* whereby communities contribute to the implementation of programmes designed by 'health experts';
- *Dialogical approaches* that seek to facilitate dialogue between health promoters and community members, developing solutions that resonate with local realities;
- *Social capital approaches* that promote participation in formal and informal networks, for example women's and youth groups; and
- Approaches having a *critical* or *political emphasis* that use community mobilization as a conduit to challenge the social inequalities that leave people vulnerable.

Favouring a mix of the dialogical and social capital approaches, with some political emphasis, Howard-Grabman and Snetro (2003) define community mobilization as a capacity-building *process* through which local individuals, groups or organizations identify needs, plan, carry out and evaluate activities on a *participatory and sustained* basis, so as *to improve health and other needs*, based on their own initiative or stimulated by others. Key characteristics of good practice that underpin community mobilization are that it should:

- Build on the already existing community processes and structures, such as health committees, or other community development initiatives;
- Develop an ongoing dialogue between community members regarding health issues;
- Create or strengthen community-based organizations aimed at improving health;
- Assist in creating an environment in which individuals can empower themselves to address their own and their community's health and other needs;
- Promote community members' participation in ways that recognize diversity and equity, especially those who are most affected by health issues;
- Work in partnership with community members in all phases of a project to create locally appropriate and locally owned responses to health needs;

- Identify and support the creative potential of communities to develop a variety of strategies and approaches to improve health status and well-being;
- Assist in linking communities with external resources (organizations, funding, technical assistance); and
- Commit enough time to work with communities, or with a partner who works with them, to accomplish the above.

Given these characteristics, and in order to design a community mobilization strategy that is feasible, acceptable, and locally appropriate, it is also good practice to include a research component at the beginning to find out about the history of the community, what has gone before, the community power dynamics, the strengths, weaknesses, and opportunities associated with – and threats to – any possible intervention.

✎ Activity 8.1

Communities are not homogeneous entities, and it is important for health promoters to define what they mean by 'community' in their community mobilization programme. This activity encourages you to reflect on the diversity of community.

1 Make a list of communities you belong to.
2 Think about what qualifies you to be a member of these communities and how each of these communities plays a role in facilitating your health and well-being.

Feedback

Your examples will show how diverse communities are, how they overlap, and how they influence behaviour. Communities tend to be tied together by having something in common. This might be a shared goal (for example, a women's group), history (for example, a group of ex-service people), belief system (for example, the Muslim community), interest or hobby (for example, football players), identity (for example, people living with HIV), or geographical space (for example, a village).

Participatory Learning and Action in community mobilization

Most health promoters looking to develop healthy communities through community mobilization draw on the Participatory Learning and Action (PLA) cycle. Guided by the works of Chambers (1983), Freire (1970), and Lewin (1946), the PLA cycle is used as a generic 'umbrella' term to describe a process whereby diverse groups and individuals come together to learn, work, and act in a cooperative manner, to focus on issues of joint concern, identify challenges, and generate positive responses in a collaborative and democratic manner. Figure 8.1 illustrates what a typical PLA cycle might look like.

There are many examples of how the PLA cycle has been adapted to community mobilization programming. This reflects the fact that there is effectively no single 'right way' to mobilize communities. However, all PLA approaches share the principle that increased knowledge can lead to action and empower communities to identify and act out solutions to local problems. Table 8.1 provides an overview of some of the ways in which a PLA approach has been used within community mobilization projects. The table demonstrates

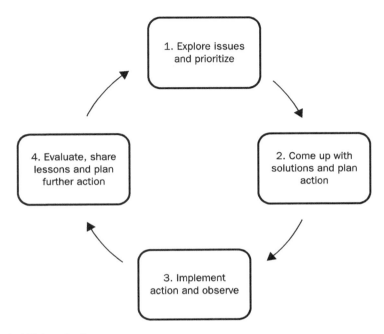

Figure 8.1 Typical PLA cycle diagram.

Table 8.1 Examples of PLA approaches to community mobilization for health

PLA approach	Description	'How to' guides
Community Action Cycles	Save the Children have developed Community Action Cycles (CAC) to describe its community mobilization programming that fosters a community-led process, through which those most affected explore, set priorities, plan, and act collectively towards better health outcomes. Steps in the CAC include preparing to mobilize; organizing for action; exploring the issues affecting access to and quality of health services and setting priorities; planning together; acting together; evaluating together; and 'scaling up' successful efforts. Each step of the CAC has a series of related activities that guide communities and facilitating partners.	Howard-Grabman and Snetro (2003)
Community Conversations	Although early versions of the Community Conversations (CC) approach have been part of development programming since the 1990s, the approach was modelled by the United Nations Development Programme (UNDP) in 2001 in their Community Capacity Enhancement Handbooks. Community Conversations provide community members with the opportunity to discuss sensitive and health-related issues. Through a series of conversations, a facilitator supports the community to identify key issues and solutions/actions that community members can take to improve health in their community.	Gueye et al. (2005)

(Continued)

Table 8.1 Continued

PLA approach	Description	'How to' guides
Women's groups	Women and Children First (UK), in collaboration with the Institute of Global Health at University College London, pioneered ways of working with women's groups to support women to identify and prioritize solutions that can address maternal, newborn, and child health problems. Groups of between 25 and 30 women meet regularly and use PLA methods to develop and implement low-tech solutions to their health problems.	Rosato *et al.* (2010)
Child-to-Child approach	The Child-to-Child (CtC) approach, developed by Professor David Morley of University College London, is an educational process that links children's learning with taking action to promote the health, well-being, and development of themselves, their families, and their communities. Through participating in Child-to-Child activities, the personal, physical, social, emotional, moral, and intellectual development of children is enhanced. The CtC methodology encourages children to work together to find solutions to real-life problems and to apply what they have learnt in their everyday lives. The children are also encouraged to share what they have learned with other children and other members of the community.	Bonati (undated)
Community-based capital cash transfers	The Ministry of Gender, Children and Social Development of Kenya, with support from the Ministry of Foreign Affairs of Denmark (DANIDA), implemented in the 1990s and 2000s a community capacity support programme (CCSP) that used PLA methods to help communities democratically prioritize problems faced by community members, identify solutions, and develop social action plans. Action plans were submitted to district level social development offices for approval and funds were transferred into community bank accounts, providing the communities with much needed capital to collectively implement their planned activities.	Skovdal *et al.* (2011)

that both community mobilization and the way in which a PLA approach can be used within these projects take many different forms.

Common to the PLA approaches is a commitment to use tools and techniques that can engage communities throughout the project cycle.

Tools, techniques, and methods to facilitate community mobilization

To help facilitate an inclusive, participatory, and empowering process whereby community members can plan, carry out, and evaluate activities that promote collective action to improve health and well-being, a number of PLA tools and techniques have been developed. In this, and the next section, we describe a range of these tools and techniques and illustrate how some of them have been used in 'real-life' programmes. The *Tools Together Now – 100 Participatory Tools to Mobilise Communities for HIV/AIDS* by the International HIV/AIDS Alliance offers a comprehensive compilation of participatory tools and techniques (International HIV/AIDS Alliance, 2006). It groups these tools and techniques into seven categories:

1 *Mapping tools* seek to develop maps that contain information about local realities and practices.
2 *Time analysis tools* focus on temporal aspects of community life, looking for example at changes over time or between seasons.
3 *Linkages and relationships tools* seek to visualize the connections between different factors promoting or undermining health.
4 *Experiential tools* seek to bring forward community members' experiences.
5 *Prioritization and quantification tools* help community members seek consensus through ranking and scoring.
6 *Action planning techniques* systematize the planning and evaluation process.
7 *Training tools* prepare facilitators to use the tools in a flexible, engaged, inclusive, and participatory way.

Examples of such tools and techniques are described below and many others are available (International HIV/AIDS Alliance, 2006).

Tool 1: Photovoice

What is Photovoice?

Photovoice is an experiential tool that enables community members, including children, to identify, represent, and enhance their community and life circumstances through photography (Wang *et al.*, 1998). Photovoice can be used to explore issues and set priorities as well as to evaluate activities.

How do you use Photovoice?

There is no single way of using Photovoice, but it might include the following steps:

1 Participants *decide on a focus* for their photography (for example, causes and consequences of malnutrition)
2 Participants move around the community for an agreed period and *take pictures*. They can either use digital cameras, including camera phones if available, or disposable cameras.
3 Participants meet up again to *write or talk about their photos*. This could involve explaining the meaning behind each photo, the reason why the photo was taken, and the relevance of the topic to people in the community.
4 Participants then share their favourite pictures and captions, and collectively the community *reflect* on the pictures taken and *identify common themes*. These themes can be used to inform health promotion activities.

Tool 2: Problem tree (explore issues and prioritize)

What is a problem tree?

A problem tree is a linkages and relationships tool. It uses the drawing of a tree, including its roots, trunk, and branches, to identify and analyse the underlying causes and the impact of an issue affecting health in the community. If, for example, after the use of another tool, such as Photovoice, diabetes was identified as a growing problem in the community, a problem tree can be used to identify the causes and effects of this problem. A problem tree can be used both to explore issues and to examine barriers to community mobilization success.

How do you use the problem tree tool?

1 Start by drawing the shape of a tree on a large piece of flipchart paper.
2 Write the issue identified by community members on the trunk of the tree (for example, diabetes).
3 By the roots of the tree encourage community members to discuss and record what they consider to be the underlying causes of this problem. For some of the main causes ask 'why do you think this might happen?' to spark debate and learning.
4 By the branches of the tree encourage community members to discuss and record the effects of this problem. Keeping with the example of diabetes, you might want to ask what the impact of this condition is for those affected, their family and friends, and other members of the community.
5 Discuss what the problem tree shows and how findings can be translated into solutions or actions.

Tool 3: Picture cards

What are picture cards?

Picture cards are a versatile tool that can be used in prioritization and quantification and in training. They are visual ways to facilitate understanding about community health issues and prioritize which issues are the most common and serious in the community. Picture cards are an especially effective tool to use with groups who have low levels of literacy. On one side of the card there is the picture, and on the other side are a series of questions the facilitator asks to prompt a group discussion about the issue.

How do you use picture cards?

1 The facilitator shows a series of 5–6 picture cards, each illustrating an issue, to the assembled group.
2 The facilitator asks questions to elicit their perceptions of the most common and serious illnesses affecting their community; the local name and connotations associated with the illness; and local practices and health actions carried out to seek care, prevent or manage the illness.
3 Through two-way dialogue the group learns correct and factual information about the issue. The facilitator is able to address negative cultural and traditional beliefs and practices in seeking health care, managing and preventing the illness.
4 The group ranks the issues that most affect their community and are the most common and serious.
5 The group choose which issue they would like to plan and take action on and vote with stones. The picture card with most stones is the health problem community members will address first.

Tool 4: Pairwise ranking

What is pairwise ranking?

Pairwise ranking is a prioritization and quantification tool that helps the community to identify preferences or priorities (Rifkin and Pridmore, 2001). In a matrix, items (for example, health problems or activities that act as solutions to health problems) are juxtaposed and community members vote on which item they wish to tackle first. The community can use this tool to prioritize and rank their preferences.

How do you use pairwise ranking?

1 Community members agree on a list of 4–8 items to be ranked. These items may be identified through another tool, such as Photovoice.
2 Draw a grid/matrix on flipchart paper with the items to be compared written at the top of the grid and again down the left-hand side (see Table 8.2).
3 Starting with the top-right square, ask participants to consider the two items and decide which one they think is more important. Compare items and record which one participants rate as most important for the remaining squares.
4 Count the preferences and rank the items.

Tool 5: Visioning how

What is visioning how?

Visioning how is an action planning tool that is used to flesh out plausible activities that could be included in an action plan. Visioning how thereby takes the health problem as prioritized by the community and maps out activities that can address this health problem.

Table 8.2 Example of pairwise ranking

Health problems	Soil-transmitted helminths	Malaria	Dengue fever	Sleeping sickness	Dysentery
Soil-transmitted helminths	—	Malaria	Soil-transmitted helminths	Soil-transmitted helminths	Dysentery
Malaria	—	—	Malaria	Malaria	Malaria
Dengue fever	—	—	—	Dengue fever	Dysentery
Sleeping sickness	—	—	—	—	Dysentery
Dysentery	—	—	—	—	—

Health problems	No. of times considered more important	Rank
Malaria	4	1
Dysentery	3	2
Soil-transmitted helminths	2	3
Dengue fever	1	4
Sleeping sickness	0	5

How do you use visioning how?

1 Ask the community members to close their eyes and take five minutes to think about what activities are likely to have the greatest impact on addressing the health issue they have decided to tackle.

2 Write a 'how' question based on the health issue the community wants to address. An example question could be: 'How can we address the problem of malaria in our community?'

3 Draw arrows coming from the 'how' question and encourage community members to give different suggestions as to how they can address the issue (for example, addressing malaria could involve increasing the use of mosquito nets). Record the different reasons by the different arrows.

4 By each of the suggested activities, draw some more arrows and explore how they will go about planning this, the resources required, etc. Record this information next to the different arrows.

5 Repeat this process until concrete plans have emerged and can be imported into an action plan.

If the community suggests many activities and needs to prioritize them, a prioritization tool can be used.

Tool 6: Action plan

What is an action plan?

An action plan is used to capture the results of the community's discussions during the PLA process, where the community carefully:

- describes the issues;
- sets priorities and specifies the objectives and desired results;
- details the activities for implementation and those responsible for implementing them;
- sets timelines.

Action plans are therefore key to the second step of the PLA cycle illustrated in Figure 8.1.

How do you develop an action plan?

A simple matrix may be used, such as the one shown in Figure 8.2. Participants may also wish to identify resources (human and material) and constraints that may help or hinder them in the pursuit of the results. The group may also want to detail the challenges that emerge from discussing the implications for implementation for each activity, and some results and activities may have to be re-evaluated and modified in the light of the challenges. Participants should decide how they are going to monitor the community's progress towards the desired results. It may be useful to design a monitoring matrix for this step, with the indicators down the left-hand side of the matrix and the following questions across the top:

- Who will be responsible for monitoring that indicator?
- How will that indicator be monitored?
- How often will it be monitored?
- What will the procedure be for reporting the monitoring results?
- What will the procedure be for reviewing and acting on the results of the monitoring?

Action Plan completed by:		Date:	
Name of clinic:		District:	
Village:		Ward:	
Problem	Actions needed	Who is responsible	When (target date)

Figure 8.2 Example of a simple action plan.

Tool 7: Log book

What is a log book?

A log book is an action planning tool that can be used to document progress in implementing an action plan. Log books can be used in the second and third steps of the PLA cycle illustrated in Figure 8.1. There may be many small sub-groups of the larger group who are implementing a variety of actions/activities at different times, which may be challenging to track for the facilitator or health committee members. A log book facilitates documentation and coordination between the main facilitator or committee members and the implementers.

How do you develop a log book?

A simple exercise book can be used by each group detailing the name of the activity being implemented, the date action took place, and progress on implementation. This information can be shared with other groups at the next community meeting and recorded on the 'master' action plan.

Tool 8: Community notice board

What is a community notice board?

A community notice board is a planning and evaluation tool, and can be used to share information and promote transparency and accountability by displaying results from activities carried out during the PLA process to the wider community (step 4 of Figure 8.1).

How do you develop a community notice board?

A notice board is positioned in a place where community members gather frequently, such as at a community centre, school, market place, health facility, district administrative headquarters or water collection point. The members of the community group regularly update the notice board, keeping the wider community informed about the activities implemented during the PLA cycle, the results of the action taken, successes, challenges, and lessons. It is hoped that sharing of information will create interest and motivate other community members to join in taking action, as well as creating a climate of accountability and transparency within the community.

✎ **Activity 8.2**

It is the role of a PLA facilitator to use tools and techniques, like the ones described above, to empower communities to explore, plan, implement, and evaluate activities that promote their health. This activity encourages you to think about what skills, knowledge, attitudes, and behaviours a PLA facilitator needs by drawing a body map. Figure 8.3 illustrates how you can use the body (as a metaphor) to map out the characteristics of a PLA facilitator.

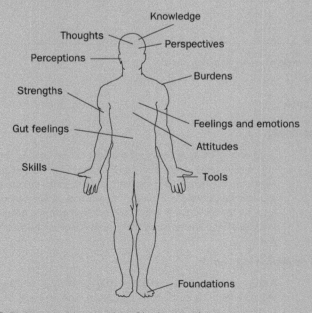

Figure 8.3 Body map with examples of body metaphors.

Draw a silhouette of a body. Use the body illustration to map out the skills, knowledge, attitudes, and behaviours a PLA facilitator needs (taking inspiration from the metaphors in Figure 8.3). Write down the knowledge, attitudes, and behaviours of a good PLA facilitator on the left side of the body, and the knowledge, attitudes, and behaviours of a poor PLA facilitator on the right of the body.

Feedback

A good PLA facilitator listens, can ask the right questions, has good interpersonal and mediation skills, is respectful, empathetic, non-judgemental, reflective of power hierarchies, inclusive, can build trust, can resolve conflicts, has in-depth knowledge of the health issue under study, can work as part of a team, has knowledge of PLA tools, is positive and enthusiastic. A poor PLA facilitator exhibits none of the above (see also example in Figure 8.4). The list above is not exhaustive and you may have identified many other qualities. The body map you have created is another example of a PLA tool.

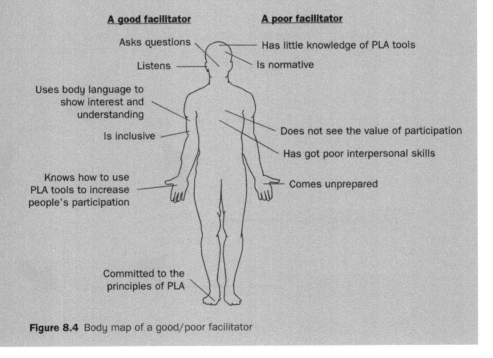

Figure 8.4 Body map of a good/poor facilitator

Case studies

To demonstrate how PLA tools can be used in practice, this chapter now describes two community mobilization programmes. The first is a large-scale programme (ACCESS) in Bangladesh and the second describes a smaller scale child-focused project in Kenya.

Case study 8.1: Community Action Cycle from Save the Children

ACCESS was a multi-country programme that was implemented in Bangladesh, Malawi, and Nigeria between 2006 and 2009. It aimed to reduce maternal and newborn deaths that result from pregnancy and childbirth complications by systematically engaging communities to improve maternal and newborn health (MNH) outcomes through Community Action Cycles, which is a tested and documented approach of community mobilization (ACCESS, 2010).

The programme's primary role was to support community mobilization for MNH by:

- Facilitating the integration of community mobilization with the broader national, regional or district health plan;
- Supporting implementing organizations (Ministry of Health, local government or non-governmental organizations [NGOs]) to develop community mobilization technical skills and expertise through training, targeted technical assistance, and joint development of guidelines, manuals, and supportive communication materials; and
- Monitoring progress of community mobilization efforts to refine strategies, energize stakeholders, and contribute to community mobilization expansion/scale-up planning.

The process described below maps out the steps taken and activities carried out to implement the ACCESS project. The phases refer to the phases of the Community Action Cycle described in Figure 8.5.

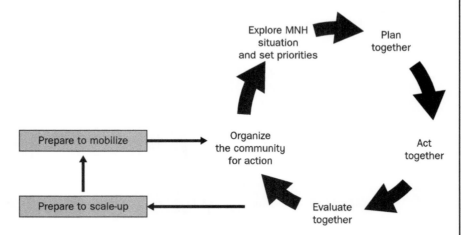

Figure 8.5 Community Action Cycle.

Preparing to mobilize phase
Step 1: Formative research was carried out in order to design a locally appropriate, context-specific community mobilization strategy for each country.

Organizing the community for action phase
Step 2: Individuals who were to facilitate the community mobilization process within communities were selected and trained.

Exploring the situation and setting priorities phase

Step 3: Activities were carried out to raise community awareness about the local MNH situation.

Step 4: Project staff worked with community leaders and other community members to invite and organize participation of those most affected by and interested in MNH.

Step 5: The facilitator explored with community members the local practices, beliefs, and attitudes that affect MNH.

Step 6: The community members were supported to set local priorities for action.

Planning together phase

Step 7: Facilitators helped community members develop and implement their own community action plans.

Acting together and evaluating together phases

Step 8: Facilitators worked with community members to build their capacity to independently monitor and evaluate their progress towards achieving improved health outcomes for mothers and newborns.

Table 8.3 summarizes the inputs and results of Community Action Cycles in Bangladesh. The development of skilled community mobilization facilitators was essential. None of the programmes provided monetary incentives to community members to organize, analyse, and address the local barriers to MNH in their communities. Those community members with heightened awareness of the problems faced by families acted collectively out of a desire to make a difference.

Table 8.3 Inputs and results matrix for the ACCESS Programme Bangladesh, February 2006 to July 2009: an NGO-led model (ACCESS, 2010)

Context	Inputs	Results
• Population covered by the intervention: approximately 795,000 • Most community health workers (CHWs) inactive and many vacant posts • Severely limited access to public, facility-based MNH services • No funding to strengthen public service delivery • Active NGO environment • Neonatal mortality rate: 37/1000 • Skilled attendance at birth: 11% • Total fertility rate: 3.7 • Modern contraceptive prevalence rate: 32%	• Community mobilization training manual, tools and communication materials developed • 125 NGO staff trained and supported to facilitate community mobilization • More than 2500 local leaders instructed on how to lead community mobilization efforts • 1904 Community Action Groups (CAGs) received monthly facilitation support • CAGs were composed of 21,875 men and women who participated to track pregnancies in their communities, and create and implement plans to encourage healthy home practices and remove barriers to use of services • 56% of CAGs included Ministry of Health staff	• 61% of CAGs generated community emergency funds (to date used by 619 families for transportation or doctors' fees, drug purchase or food) • 83% of CAGs organized emergency transport systems (to date used by 436 mothers and 247 newborns) for cases of obstructed labour, retained placenta, convulsions and (in the newborn) pneumonia, convulsions and jaundice, among others • CAGs re-opened 69 inactive clinics and EPI centres, and opened 12 new satellite clinics and 2 EPI centres, working closely with local government and NGO representatives

✎ **Activity 8.3**

When designing large-scale community mobilization projects, it is important to think about what will be left after the project has ended at all levels of engagement (community, district, national levels).

1 How can you promote sustainability and ownership at all levels of the project?
2 How can you ensure that communities continue to take action over a sustained period?
3 How can you ensure the project reaches the most vulnerable and marginalized for a sustained period of time?

Feedback

- When designing your project, you will need to use formative research and pre-testing of concepts with the different levels of stakeholder to gauge what will motivate communities to engage over a sustained period.
- Research should look at: community power dynamics (for example, existing structures and opportunities); decision-makers and gatekeepers (for example, community and religious leaders); volunteer motivation and non-financial incentives (for example, for facilitators and participants, such as status, collective identity, respect); stakeholder analysis, power mapping, and consultation at higher levels to gain buy-in.
- The capacity-building of local non-governmental organizations (NGOs), civil society organizations (CSOs), and community-based organizations (CBOs), and their ability as partners to engage with community members over a longer period of time, can ensure that the most vulnerable and marginalized are reached (for example, organizations working with people living with HIV and disability; women's groups; children's clubs).

Case study 8.2: Strengthening the coping strategies of young carers in western Kenya

This community mobilization project was initiated by a local NGO in western Kenya in order to strengthen the coping and resilience of children caring for their sick parents or elderly grandparents (Skovdal, 2010). The project was made up of six PLA steps and engaged two rural, low-resource, and high-HIV prevalence communities.

Step 1 involved sensitizing the communities to the project and recruiting young carers. In partnership with community health workers, 48 young carers from the two communities were identified and invited to participate in the project. The young carers were aged 12–17 years.

Step 2 involved getting the young carers together in their respective communities (24 children from each community), introducing them to each other, to the NGO, and the aim of the project. To establish group dynamics, the young carers were provided with sports equipment and drawing materials and encouraged to meet up regularly.

Step 3 involved facilitating a number of participatory learning and action workshops to help the children identify and discuss their strengths, local coping resources and struggles. This involved using Photovoice (see above). After some training on how to use the disposable cameras they were given and the ethics of taking pictures, the children took photos, over a two-week period, guided by the following four questions:

- What is your life like?
- What is good about your life?
- What makes you strong?
- What needs to change?

When the children returned and all the photographs had been developed, they were invited to pick six of their favourite photographs, showing a mix of how they get by, things they lack, and something or someone who is important to them. They were then asked to reflect and write a story about each of their chosen photographs, prompted by the following questions:

- I want to share this photo because . . .
- What's the real story this photo tells?
- How does this story relate to your life and/or the lives of people in your community?

If the children wanted to write about a situation that they did not capture on camera, for ethical or practical reasons, they were encouraged to draw the situation.

Step 4 involved the young carers sharing their stories and observations from these participatory learning activities, identifying common struggles and coping strategies. Through prioritization tools, such as pairwise ranking and action planning techniques, the young carers drew on the themes emerging from their reflections and photos to decide on a list of activities to include in an action plan. Each of the two groups of young carers developed an action plan that would strengthen their coping and resilience. Both groups felt that they could benefit from learning how to run a small-scale enterprise. One of the groups of young carers therefore decided to engage in goat and chicken rearing and farming, while the other group decided to set up a small business selling corn.

Step 5 involved the NGO funding the action plans developed by the two groups of young carers and supporting them to implement the activities. This included providing the young carers with the necessary training to run a small-scale enterprise and conducting frequent visits to support and offer advice where required.

Step 6 involved evaluating progress of their activities. The young carers were invited to write a story about 'being part of a team', guided by the following three questions:

- What are your feelings about being part of a team?
- What, if anything, have you learnt from being part of a team?
- Why do you think that is?

The young carers were also invited to draw and write about their experiences. More specifically, they were encouraged to draw and write about: (i) the activities they implemented; (ii) those who were involved; (iii) a situation where they faced a problem. The essays and drawings were shared among the young carers in workshops, sparking debate about what they had learned and how they were able, as a collective, to overcome difficulties as they move forward.

Evidence on the effectiveness of community mobilization

Much has been written about community mobilization over the years and many lessons have been learnt from community mobilization programmes in both low-income and high-income countries. Although the evidence is mixed, the health-promoting potential of community mobilization programming is promising. This is demonstrated by a growing number of successful, tried-and-tested approaches to community mobilization. In the context of maternal, newborn, and child health, for example, researchers from the Institute of Global Health at University College London, have developed and tested an approach that involves training local female facilitators to establish women's groups and support a participatory and action-oriented process that strengthens the capacity of women in the community to take control of their health and that of their children (Prost *et al.*, 2013). The researchers found the application of this low-cost, scalable, and participatory model improves birth outcomes in a poor rural populations in Nepal (Manandhar *et al.*, 2004), India (Tripathy *et al.*, 2010), Bangladesh (Azad *et al.*, 2010), and Malawi (Lewycka *et al.*, 2013). There is also evidence that community mobilization efforts taken to scale have achieved significant health gains. For example, in Ethiopia a cluster randomized controlled trial showed that mobilizing women's groups to effectively recognize and treat malaria at home led to a 40% reduction in under-5 mortality (Kidane and Morrow, 2000). In Bolivia, as part of the Warmi project, women's groups, led by a locally recruited woman facilitator, and supported through a community mobilization action cycle, discussed maternal and newborn health problems. Strategies were developed, implemented, and assessed in cooperation with local leaders, men, and health workers. The project saw a 30% reduction in the neonatal mortality rate (O'Rourke *et al.*, 1998). A recent systematic review by Cornish *et al.* (2014) also demonstrates the potential of community mobilization in the context of HIV prevention.

Mobile technologies and social media are changing the social landscape and communication between people and organizations across the globe, offering new and exciting opportunities for community mobilization. The potential of mobile technologies to take the principles of community mobilization (i.e. facilitate critical awareness and empower people to push for change) to an unprecedented scale is set to transform health and development services globally (Zambrano and Seward, 2012). Future community mobilization programmes ought to harness current advances in mobile technology in community mobilization, both to enable people to challenge and address the social inequalities that leave them vulnerable in the first place, and to better engage with people in urban zones and areas with migratory and transient populations.

Challenges, uses, and abuses of community mobilization

While there are many examples of community mobilization strategies that have been successful in improving health outcomes throughout the world, not all community mobilization programmes succeed. Community mobilization is a process that depends on the interpersonal skills and attitudes of the stakeholders involved. To help circumvent and prepare for some of the many challenges related to community mobilization, this chapter now outlines some common pitfalls.

- *Power relations* – it is important to be aware of the power relationships within a community. Communities experience power dynamics and politics that are difficult for outside facilitators to understand. Be aware of gender dynamics; the sensitivity of certain topics; tensions between old and young; feuds between families and neighbours; the role of community leaders; difficulties in agreeing on community priorities and planned actions, responsibilities, and timescales.

- *Capacity-building* – care should be taken not to underestimate the need for capacity-building. Inadequate support and training can lead to community apathy, frustration, and demotivation, resulting in inaction. Equally, capacity-building activities should not assume that community members have no knowledge or experience to incorporate and build on.
- *Time commitments* – community mobilization is a time-consuming process, requiring commitment from both the facilitating agency and from community members. For community members, volunteering time can be a challenge, and some community members may feel overstretched and burdened by the process.

In addition to recognizing some of the challenges inherent to community mobilization, health promoters facilitating community mobilization projects need to be aware of the risk of more powerful stakeholders hijacking and taking advantage of what community mobilization projects can offer, or in some cases, disguise, in order to support their own agenda. Potential 'uses and abuses' (cf. White, 1996; Cooke and Kothari, 2001; Mosse, 2001) of community mobilization to be aware of include:

- *'Facipulation'* – this terms describes the process by which community mobilization can be used as a guise to manipulate participants in a particular direction. In particular, the process of facilitating community mobilization can be steered and guided to different degrees and in different ways, with the risk that some community mobilization projects may be 'facipulated' to convince local people of the agendas of others.
- *Appropriateness* – it is possible that community mobilization and participation may carry more significance for health promoters than it does for the communities participating. This is particularly the case where challenging power relations and the status quo may be detrimental to the community and may leave them more vulnerable, marginalized, and exposed in some hostile environments.
- *Cheap solution* – despite the health promotion potential of community mobilization, it is not the responsibility of community members to substitute the role and responsibilities of health institutions and structures. Community mobilization should therefore not be used as a justification for avoiding necessary health and welfare spending or seen as a cheaper goal than reducing income inequalities.

Despite these challenges and potential 'uses and abuses', community mobilization continues to be ethically and practically fundamental to developing health-enabling community contexts.

✏ Activity 8.4

In this activity you will conduct a Strengths, Weaknesses, Opportunities, Threats (SWOT) analysis of a programme looking to develop healthy communities through community mobilization.

EITHER re-visit one of the two community mobilization programme case studies above to do this hypothetically, OR think of a community mobilization programme you are familiar with. Consider the strengths, weaknesses, opportunities, and threats of the programme by completing a SWOT diagram (as illustrated in Figure 8.6). Strengths and weaknesses refer to internal factors facilitating or inhibiting the programme, while opportunities and threats refer to external factors.

		Facilitators	Barriers
Internal factors		Strengths	Weaknesses
External factors		Opportunities	Threats

Figure 8.6 SWOT diagram.

Feedback

Through this process you should have identified both internal and external factors serving as either barriers or facilitators in achieving the objective of community mobilization activities. Figure 8.7 highlights what some of the factors might be.

		Facilitators	Barriers
Internal factors		**Strengths** • The quality of the PLA facilitator • Programme planning • Capacity-building • Partnership between agency and community	**Weaknesses** • Poor leadership • Elements of facipulation • Limited time available
External factors		**Opportunities** • Use of new mobile technologies • Integration of activities into health services • National policies • Community mobilization is valued by stakeholders	**Threats** • Power imbalances within the community • Weather (such as drought) • Funding is limited or cut short • Conflict

Figure 8.7 Potential strengths, weaknesses, opportunities, and threats.

Summary

This chapter has introduced you to community mobilization and offered a series of tools and approaches that can help you build healthy communities through community mobilization. More specifically, you have learnt about the PLA cycle and how it can be flexibly adapted to different contexts, as long as it offers community members the opportunity to develop a critical perspective about their health needs and the chance to develop community-driven responses. You have been introduced to specific tools and methods for facilitating participatory learning and action, and seen how these tools can be applied in both small- and large-scale community mobilization programmes. You have also covered some of the potential challenges and 'uses and abuses' of community mobilization programmes.

References

ACCESS (March 2010) *Community Mobilization: An Effective Strategy to Improve MNH, Household-to-Hospital Continuum of Maternal and Newborn Care*. Baltimore, MD: JHPIEGO/USAID.

Azad, K., Barnett, S., Banerjee, B., Shaha, S., Khan, K., Rego, A.R. et al. (2010) Effect of scaling up women's groups on birth outcomes in three rural districts in Bangladesh: a cluster-randomised controlled trial, *The Lancet*, 375 (9721): 1193–1202.

Bonati, G. (undated) *Child-to-Child and Vulnerable Children: Supporting Vulnerable Children Using the Child-to-Child Approach*. London/Brighton: ProVIC/International HIV/AIDS Alliance/Child-to-Child [http://www.child-to-child.org/resources/pdfs/Manual-C2C-Vulnerable Children.pdf; accessed 4 September 2014].

Campbell, C. (2014) Community mobilization in the 21st century: updating our theory of social change?, *Journal of Health Psychology*, 19 (1): 46–59.

Chambers, R. (1983) *Rural Development: Putting the Last First*. London: Longman.

Cooke, B. and Kothari, U. (2001) *Participation: The New Tyranny?* London: Zed Books.

Cornish, F., Priego-Hernandez, J., Campbell, C., Mburu, G. and McLean, S. (2014) The impact of community mobilization on HIV prevention in middle and low income countries: a systematic review and critique, *AIDS and Behavior*, 18: 2110–34.

Freire, P. (1970) *Pedagogy of the Oppressed*. London: Penguin Books.

Gueye, M., Diouf, D., Chaava, T. and Tiomkin, D. (2005) *Community Capacity Enhancement Strategy Note: The Answer Lies Within*. New York: United Nations Development Programme.

Howard-Grabman, L. and Snetro, G. (2003) *How to Mobilize Communities for Health and Social Change*. Baltimore, MD: Health Communication Partnership/USAID [http://www.jhuccp.org/resource_center/publications/field_guides_tools/how-mobilize-communities-health-and-social-change-20; accessed 14 April 2014].

International HIV/AIDS Alliance (2006) *Tools Together Now: 100 Participatory Tools to Mobilise Communities for HIV/AIDS*. Brighton: International HIV/AIDS Alliance [http://www.aidsalliance.org/assets/000/000/370/229-Tools-together-now_original.pdf?1405520036; accessed 14 April 2014].

Kidane, G. and Morrow, R.H. (2000) Teaching mothers to provide home treatment of malaria in Tigray, Ethiopia: a randomised trial, *The Lancet*, 356 (9229): 550–5.

Lewin, K. (1946) Action research and minority problems, *Journal of Social Issues*, 2 (4): 34–46.

Lewycka, S., Mwansambo, C., Rosato, M., Kazembe, P., Phiri, T., Mganga, A. et al. (2013) Effect of women's groups and volunteer peer counselling on rates of mortality, morbidity, and health behaviours in mothers and children in rural Malawi (MaiMwana): a factorial, cluster-randomised controlled trial, *The Lancet*, 381 (9879): 1721–35.

Manandhar, D.S., Osrin, D., Shrestha, B.P., Mesko, N., Morrison, J., Tumbahangphe, K.M. et al. (2004) Effect of a participatory intervention with women's groups on birth outcomes in Nepal: cluster-randomised controlled trial, *The Lancet*, 364 (9438): 970–9.

Mosse, D. (2001) 'People's participation', participation and patronage: operations and representations in rural development, in B. Cooke and U. Kothari (eds.) *Participation: The New Tyranny?* (pp. 17–35). London: Zed Books.

O'Rourke, K., Howard-Grabman, L. and Seoane, G. (1998) Impact of community organization of women on perinatal outcomes in rural Bolivia, *Revista Panamericana de Salud Pública*, 3 (1): 9–14.

Prost, A., Colbourn, T., Seward, N., Azad, K., Coomarasamy, A., Copas, A. *et al.* (2013) Women's groups practising participatory learning and action to improve maternal and newborn health in low-resource settings: a systematic review and meta-analysis, *The Lancet*, 381 (9879): 1736–46.

Rifkin, S. and Pridmore, P. (2001) *Partners in Planning: Information, Participation and Empowerment*. London: TALC/Macmillan Education.

Rosato, M., Mwansambo, C., Lewycka, S., Kazembe, P., Phiri, T., Malamba, F. *et al.* (2010) MaiMwana women's groups: a community mobilization intervention to improve mother and child health and reduce mortality in rural Malawi, *Malawi Medical Journal*, 22 (4): 112–19.

Skovdal, M. (2010) Community relations and child-led microfinance: a case study of caregiving children in Western Kenya, *AIDS Care*, 22 (suppl. 2): 1652–61.

Skovdal, M. (2013) Using theory to guide change at the community level, in L. Cragg, M. Davies and W. Macdowall (eds.) Health Promotion Theory (2nd edn., pp. 79–97). Maidenhead: Open University Press.

Skovdal, M., Mwasiaji, W., Webale, A. and Tomkins, A. (2011) Building orphan competent communities: experiences from a community-based capital cash transfer initiative in Kenya, *Health Policy and Planning*, 26 (3): 233–41.

Tripathy, P., Nair, N., Barnett, S., Mahapatra, R., Borghi, J., Rath, S. *et al.* (2010) Effect of a participatory intervention with women's groups on birth outcomes and maternal depression in Jharkhand and Orissa, India: a cluster-randomised controlled trial, *The Lancet*, 375 (9721): 1182–92.

Wang, C., Yi, W., Tao, Z. and Carovano, K. (1998) Photovoice as a participatory health promotion strategy, *Health Promotion International*, 13 (1): 75–86.

White, S. (1996) Depoliticising development: the uses and abuses of participation, *Development in Practice*, 6: 6–15.

World Health Organization (WHO) (1978) *Declaration of Alma-Ata*. Geneva: WHO [http://www.who.int/publications/almaata_declaration_en.pdf].

World Health Organization (WHO) (1986) *Ottawa Charter for Health Promotion*. Geneva: WHO [http://www.who.int/healthpromotion/conferences/previous/ottawa/en/].

World Health Organization (WHO) (2005) *Bangkok Charter for Health Promotion*. Geneva: WHO [http://www.who.int/healthpromotion/conferences/6gchp/hpr_050829_%20BCHP.pdf].

Zambrano, R. and Seward, R. (2012) *Mobile Technologies and Empowerment: Enhancing Human Development through Participation and Innovation*. New York: United Nations Development Programme [http://issuu.com/undp/docs/mobile_technologies_and_empowerment_en; accessed 12 May 2014].

Further reading

Howard-Grabman, L. and Snetro, G. (2003) *How to Mobilize Communities for Health and Social Change*. Baltimore, MD: Health Communication Partnership/USAID [http://www.jhuccp.org/resource_center/publications/field_guides_tools/how-mobilize-communities-health-and-social-change-20; accessed 14 April 2014].

Using media to promote health: mass media, social media, and social marketing

9

Will Nutland

Overview

This chapter explores how different media are used within health promotion. First, the chapter examines the more traditional ways of delivering health promotion using mass media, and discusses the advantages and disadvantages of using mass media to influence health. The emergence of social media, and its proliferation in the field of public health and health promotion, is then explored and how its use might add to or detract from the influence of other media methods on health. Finally, the chapter discusses the role of social marketing within health promotion, outlining the key stages of developing a social marketing intervention in practice, and considers if a marketing approach can also be used to 'market' health.

Learning objectives

After reading this chapter, you will be able to:

- describe the strengths and limitations of using mass media in health promotion practice
- understand a range of different methods of using mass media and how these different methods might be applied to different target groups in health promotion practice
- compare and contrast mass media and social media methods and the relative merits of each
- explain the opportunities and challenges that the emergence and development of social media brings to delivering health promotion
- understand the key stages in the development of a social marketing intervention
- describe the challenges and complexities of using social marketing to influence health

Key terms

Audience segmentation: Identifying who is to be targeted by an intervention according to their personal characteristics, past behaviour, and the benefits they seek.

Customer orientation: A marketing term for understanding aspects of people's lives such as their characteristics, needs, and desires.

Mass media: Print and electronic channels through which information is transmitted to a large number of people at a time.

> **Social marketing**: A discipline that takes the concepts of commercial marketing and applies those concepts to influence the social beliefs and behaviours of a target audience.
>
> **Social media**: Media that enables interaction and exchange of information between those generating the content and those interacting with it.

Introduction

The mass media is one of the most commonly used ways of communicating health information to target audiences. Through public health broadcasts on radio and television; health information on billboards and public transport; adverts in magazines, newspapers, and online; and health adverts conveyed by mobile phones and other handheld devices, most people throughout the world receive some health promotion information through mass media methods.

New social media have fundamentally changed how people relate to and interact with health information. Although the World Wide Web has been in existence since the end of the twentieth century, it is only since the introduction and proliferation of social network sites, coupled with the availability of new technology such as smart phones, that social media has begun to play an important and growing part in how health information is communicated. Despite the growth of social media, little is known about the extent to which it can be used to influence health (Korda and Itani, 2013), or if it offers substantial and additional benefits to more traditional mass media methods.

Social marketing draws upon principles of traditional marketing and applies those principles to the 'marketing' of health. Social marketing is often mistakenly conflated purely with mass media or is seen as social mass media. Although social marketing has traditionally drawn on mass media, it is not purely a mass media intervention. Instead, good social marketing draws on a mix of methods, including those discussed in other chapters in this book, such as therapeutic methods, and information and advice methods. However, in reality, much health-focused social marketing draws on mass media and social media methods. For this reason, social marketing is discussed within this chapter.

The chapter addresses mass media, social media, and social marketing in turn.

Mass media

What is mass media and how is it used in health promotion?

Mass media includes television, radio, billboards, and print media such as newspapers and magazines. Information campaigns that use mass media are a common way of undertaking health promotion and have been used throughout the world. Examples include interventions to increase vaccination rates, to highlight the benefits of breastfeeding, to reduce traffic accidents, and to promote healthier lifestyles. Mass media interventions usually involve developing and placing health promotion information in appropriate text-based and audio or visual media. It is best practice for media interventions to be pre-tested to ensure that they are appropriate to, and understandable by, the target audience. Media interventions are often part of a broader health campaign that might include advertising, alongside small media, or radio or television broadcast or websites, often in conjunction with face-to-face information and advice. In this way, various media placements complement each other, and increase recognition in the target audience.

In recent decades, developments such as the internet and mobile phone technology have opened up new forms of mass media which offer potential new channels for delivering health promotion. The proliferation and availability of those technologies, at ever cheaper cost, have widened the reach of health promotion information beyond that achieved by more traditional mass media, such as billboards and radio adverts. Both the internet and mobile phone technology have dramatically changed how communication is conducted throughout the world.

However, despite its popularity, the widespread use of mass media as a health promotion method remains controversial. It has been argued that mass media can be seen as the 'easy choice' for politicians who want to be seen to be doing something to address public health, while failing to address the root causes of ill health. As mass media interventions, by definition, are seen by a broad audience, they have been criticized for being unfocused, untargeted, and having little impact on key target populations who may not encounter the media intervention. As such, they can be seen as a poor use of limited health budgets that detract resources away from community level or individual level interventions. Green and Tones (2010) have argued that many mass communications are seeking to 'sell' health, rather than increase choice and empower individuals to make their own choices, and are therefore ethically questionable. Others have voiced concerns that mass media health promotion interventions tend to focus on individual behaviour change, rather than addressing the barriers to health-seeking behaviour, and as such can result in victim-blaming. For example, a media campaign that tells its audience to wash their hands, without addressing the unavailability of washing facilities, could lead to blaming those who become unwell for not heeding the campaign's didactic instructions.

✏ Activity 9.1

Consider what you have heard, seen or read in recent weeks that contained information about health in different mass media.

Feedback

You will notice that a broad range of mass media is used to convey health information. Maybe you noticed a billboard promoting road safety, e-cigarettes, weight loss or cosmetic surgery; perhaps a radio play or TV soap opera tackling domestic violence or the benefits of vaccination; maybe you noticed cancer awareness information on posters at a health centre, or in a magazine in the waiting area; you may have seen a banner advert or a pop-up advert when you went online; or perhaps you noticed a newspaper article featuring a dance and exercise class for elders, or a feature in an online news site about the impact of poor housing on health.

Mass media and norm functioning

Despite the criticisms of mass media, it has a powerful norming function and socialization effect. The examples identified in Activity 9.1 illustrate the myriad ways that health information is generated and transmitted through mass media. Some of the examples clearly have a purposeful intention to impact on health by attempting to increase knowledge, improve access to services or change behaviour. Yet not all of the examples have a health-driven agenda and the health impact may be considered to be an 'incidental by-product' when the real goal is to increase sales of a product or to increase viewing figures. The subtle difference between health promotion advertising and commercial advertising under the guise of health promotion can be confusing for consumers and, arguably, some of the examples might appear to have a health-driven agenda (such as e-cigarettes or cosmetic surgery or weight loss products) but could be said to be buying in to social fashion of what it is to be 'healthy'. However, both the 'purposeful' and the 'incidental' impacts of mass media are important.

Finnegan and Viswanath (1997) identify that the role of mass media in health falls into two categories. The first of these is the impact of ongoing interaction with the media on health outcomes. Research has explored the influence of media consumption on attitudes and behaviours, and the influence of media portrayal of health issues on how audiences view those health issues (a process sometimes known as 'norm-sending'). Given the importance of mass media as a source of information, health promoters sometimes engage with journalists and media producers to influence how health issues are addressed within the media. This influencing of norm-sending can occur through attempting to direct contemporary public health issues in the news (for example, by 'briefing' a journalist about a health story) as well as by attempting to influence content of fictional TV and radio drama.

The second role proposed by Finnegan and Viswanath (1997) is the purposive use of the mass media to achieve a particular health outcome. More traditionally, this has involved the placement of adverts on TV, radio or in print media with the aim of increasing health knowledge, attitudes or behaviours. More recently, the methods of using mass media to convey messages have developed and expanded, including media advocacy (as is discussed in Chapter 6) and by finding more innovative ways of delivering information through radio, television, and online.

The strengths and limitations of mass media

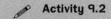 **Activity 9.2**

This chapter has outlined some of the common critiques of using mass media in health promotion. In addition to those critiques, identify what might be the strengths and the limitations of using mass media in health promotion.

Feedback

Read through the following paragraphs to see how many of the strengths and the limitations associated with using mass media in health promotion you identified.

One of the key strengths of mass media is its potential reach: print media or TV or radio adverts will have a reach that extends beyond the capacity of outreach interventions or other face-to-face interventions. Another strength is that if the media intervention is not in an outdoor setting, those who encounter the intervention can do so in their own time and space, without being concerned that others are witnessing their encounter with the intervention.

Although, on their own, mass media interventions cannot be expected to result in behaviour change, they can be an essential part of an environment in which health needs can be addressed. For example, they can be useful in raising awareness of, and signposting to, other more tailored and targeted health promotion interventions for those who encounter them.

Careful planning and placement can ensure that mass media interventions reach a clearly articulated target group. This might be through placement of adverts in magazines or newspapers read by a particular population group (such as magazines for young women); purchasing internet banner adverts on specific websites (such as a regional news site for people in a specific geographical area); running radio adverts on stations targeted at specific groups (such as a station listened to by a particular ethnic group in a region or country); or by placing adverts in venues likely to be encountered by a specific target group (such as people using a social venue where smoking, alcohol or recreational drug use occurs). Thoughtful targeting of media interventions can also make them more cost-effective.

Conversely, there is a danger that those for whom it is not intended encounter the intervention. If the health issue is relatively benign, then this might not be a concern. However, if the media intervention concerns a health issue that holds a level of taboo within some populations, then there is the danger of increasing stigma or discrimination for the intended target group. In some instances, this might put the target group in danger or at risk (for example, advertising the venue where a needle exchange programme takes place, or where an alcohol or drug service is situated).

Another limitation of mass media interventions is that they assume that the target group has access to, can afford, is able to understand, and is able to encounter the intervention in the setting in which the intervention is placed. For example, only those who have access to television sets, a reliable power supply, and those who understand the language in which the advert is spoken or written will easily be able to encounter TV adverts as they were intended. Similarly, a printed health advert will only be encountered by people with access to the publication in which it is placed (or those who pass by the static billboard or poster on which it is posted), and who are literate enough to read and understand the content.

Although placement of mass media interventions can be relatively cheap if measured against the number of people who encounter them, the total cost of development, pre-testing, design, and placement can be quite high. These costs need to be factored into the planning of an intervention.

Finally, most traditional media methods, unlike face-to-face information and advice methods, involve no interaction between the health promoter and the target audience, meaning that the information is one-directional and cannot be tailored to the specific needs of individuals. This limitation is discussed in the section below on social media.

What evidence is there to support mass media interventions?

As we have seen, mass media interventions have the potential to increase knowledge and to raise awareness among large numbers of people. They also have the potential to reach people who would not encounter other face-to-face interventions. They can have a role in presenting role models and attempting to change normative beliefs, and can assist in pushing particular health issues up the agendas of policy-makers and politicians (Wellings and Macdowall, 2000). This chapter now explores evidence from research on how effective mass media interventions are in practice.

An exploratory review of HIV mass media interventions targeting men who have sex with men (MSM) (French *et al.*, 2014) found that intervention awareness among the target group of interventions reviewed was variable and that recall of key messages was poor. The review found a lack of rigorous evidence for any significant effect of mass media interventions on MSM, although there were some short-term effects on HIV testing. Although some mass media interventions can contribute to increasing knowledge in a target group, the review concludes they are less effective in addressing motivation and skills. And, although they can set the context in which norms can be changed and stigma might be challenged, mass media interventions cannot change these factors alone. As such, mass media interventions that raise awareness and increase knowledge might be better off delivered alongside other more in-depth motivational and skills-building interventions (including those that the media intervention can direct the audience towards).

While mass media interventions have the capacity to reach a broad audience, questions remain as to whether the most commonly used methods reach those in most need of health promotion interventions. It makes sense that those with the greatest capacity to encounter mass media interventions, whether through the ability to purchase the media in which it is encountered or the ability to read or understand health promotion information, are those who are most likely to encounter the intervention itself. A study of Ethiopian media use and HIV knowledge (Bekalu and Eggermont, 2013) found that although HIV-related media use did not have a significant effect on HIV knowledge across the total population, knowledge was higher in those who were more highly educated. However, the study did find that the knowledge gap between those with higher and lower educational levels diminished as media use increased. The authors suggest that mass media interventions have the capacity to act as a 'knowledge leveller' between educational status and socio-economic status. In describing the differences between urban and rural populations' use of HIV-related health promotion media, the authors also highlight the issue of information salience – that is, the extent to which the HIV information being broadcast might be perceived as being more appealing or relevant to urban rather than rural populations. This highlights the complexity of broadcasting 'one-size-fits-all' mass media interventions. The authors suggest that a widening information gap between urban and rural communities might be addressed by delivering community-based HIV programmes and interpersonal communication activities that tap into existing social, cultural, and religious networks.

Social media

What is social media and how is it used in health promotion?

In recent years, social media has been increasingly used as a vehicle for health promotion. Unlike traditional mass media, where opportunities for interaction between the provider and recipient of the media are limited, social media enables interaction and exchange of information between those generating the content and those interacting with it. With the rapid development and accompanying relative fall in price of mobile phones and other hand-held technology, the availability and quantity of social media and the number of people who create, encounter, and engage with it has proliferated. Mobile social media technology has the added function of location-sensitivity: identifying the location of the device's user and tailoring information to those within a distinct geographical area.

Social media, or Web 2.0, is a range of technological innovations that have emerged from the first expansion in global use of the internet:

'Web 2.0' . . . refers to a loose collection of web-based technologies and services that allow end users to interact and collaborate as content creators, rather than the one-way information flow on relatively static 'Web 1.0' websites. The term 'social media' is used interchangeably with Web 2.0 to describe sites and applications that allow information sharing and interactive activities among online communities; examples include blogs, wikis, content-sharing sites, virtual worlds and social networking sites. (Gold et al., 2012)

An emphasis on user involvement has resulted in the label of the 'participative internet' (Korda and Itana, 2013). This participatory dimension of users also creating content sets social media apart from other traditional forms of media, such as television, film, and websites, that display information. However, just because an intervention is encountered online, it is not necessarily social media. For example, a website that contains static information that a user cannot interact with is not social media: it is a website.

Developments in social media have provided the potential to even small-scale health promotion organizations and projects to reach, and engage with, a wider audience. Social media sites such as Facebook have provided a structure for organizations to promote their services, and for users of the service to engage directly with the service – and other service users. Twitter has allowed for cheap and swift promotion of events. YouTube has enabled peer-driven health promotion interventions to be developed at almost no cost. Social media apps have also changed the face of service promotion – for example, apps that capture key demographics of their users can target specific adverts by such characteristics as gender or age. And apps can use geographical location to invite subscribers to attend geographically based services. This media has provided the potential for a democratization of health promotion methods.

The rise of social media in public health

Social media has rapidly become a central feature of daily life across the world and, relatedly, is seen as having a key role in health promotion (Chou et al., 2012).

 Activity 9.3

From your recent personal or professional experience, identify the benefits of using social media, rather than traditional mass media methods, to undertake health promotion.

Feedback

Commentators have suggested a range of attributes that could make social media a powerful tool for health promotion. You might have identified some of these. They include:

- The ability of social media to reach marginal groups;
- The potential low cost of social media compared with other media methods, especially given that the structure of most social media used for health promotion already exist and do not have to be created;
- The ability to tailor messages to specific audiences using social media;
- The ability of social media to provide information in safe and private spaces.

The feedback to Activity 9.3 outlines some of the potential attributes of social media that make it especially useful for delivering health promotion. However, there is, as yet, a shortage of analysis that demonstrates social media can actually achieve this potential. This partly reflects the fact that social media has emerged only recently, so there has not yet been sufficient time for research findings on its medium- and long-term impact to emerge. However, across current available research, there is little overall evidence of the efficacy of social media for promoting health (Korda and Itana, 2013). There is increasing understanding of the way in which social media can be used for particular health areas (Gold *et al.*, 2011) and the acceptability, or not, of using social media in this way to reach specific groups, such as adolescents (Byron *et al.*, 2013). However, there is still little understanding of the impact of social media interventions in health promotion on health outcomes. This lack of knowledge of the impact stands in contrast with the ever-increasing policy attention and financial and human resources being dedicated to social media within public health.

Theoretical explanations for the impact of social media on health

In addition to the paucity of evidence on the impact of social media interventions on health outcomes, there is a lack of theoretical clarity about the precise pathways that health-focused social media interventions could use to impact on knowledge and behaviour. The policy field is instead characterized by implicit or undeveloped assumptions. Theoretical frameworks used in health promotion more broadly have been suggested as useful; general frameworks such as empowerment sit alongside more specific theoretical notions of social learning theory, social cognitive theory, theories of reasoned action, and script theory (Collins *et al.*, 2010). Any evaluation frameworks are in their early stages of development (Collins *et al.*, 2010) and require further research.

Considerations for using social media in health promotion practice

As more health promotion activity is being undertaken through social media, health promotion practitioners need to continue to evaluate their social media practice and add to the body of evidence, and good practice, as interventions and innovations develop further. A systematic review of Web 2.0 for health promotion highlighted three emerging critical themes to inform future practice (Chou *et al.*, 2012):

1 *The need to harness the participatory nature of social media* – the authors highlighted the failure of most social media interventions to make the most of the unique opportunities that social media provide: namely, the ability of participants to enhance health interventions. Indeed, they discovered that in some instances in particular health issues, user participation led to stigmatization and teasing, rather than enhancing health outcomes.
2 *Information and accuracy* – the authors found that user-generated content on social media was often inconsistent with more formal health guidance and advice. They note that this offers an opportunity for health promoters to engage with and discuss misinformation or inaccurate information. Moreover, they noted the potential opportunity for dissemination of guidelines or evidence-based health information through a combination of system-generated content and user- and peer-related content that relates to an individual's experience of a health issue.
3 *Implications for the digital divide* – the authors noted the oft-cited commentaries of the potential of social media to reach marginalized populations and reduce health disparit-

ies. They note that this is not being evidenced in practice and suggest that interventions address factors such as literacy, relevance, and trust of the information source. They also note that inequitable internet access increases the divide between those who are able to and those who are unable to benefit from social media interventions.

Social marketing

What is social marketing and how is it used in health promotion?

Social marketing is a discipline that takes the concepts of commercial marketing and applies them to influence the social beliefs and behaviours of a target audience. It has been defined as 'a large scale programme planning process designed to influence the voluntary behaviour of a specific audience segment to achieve a social rather than a financial objective and based upon offering benefits the audience wants, reducing barriers the audience faces, and/or using persuasion to influence the segment's intentions to act favourably' (Albrecht, 1996: 21).

Social marketing began to be more widely applied to health promotion practice in the 1980s and at the start of the twenty-first century social marketing approaches were embedded in government health policies, including in Australia, Canada, New Zealand, the UK, and the USA.

The concept of social marketing, developed by Kotler and Zaltman (1971), works on the premise that, in the same manner as purchasing goods and services, people weigh up the costs and benefits of behaviours such as donating blood, saving energy or recycling, applying sunscreen, using a mosquito net or eating healthily. Social marketing focuses on the positive outcomes (the benefits) of changing behaviour rather than on the negative outcomes (the costs) of not altering behaviours. Social marketing is rooted in the concepts of exchange theory: that people will act out of their own self-interest to optimize the value of doing (or not doing) something that gives them the greatest benefit for the least cost. As such, a social marketing approach must first of all offer benefits to the consumer that they strongly value and, secondly, recognize the costs associated with changing behaviour.

Social marketing in practice

Social marketing practitioners commonly use a five-stage model of social marketing development: scoping, development, implementation, evaluation, and follow-up.

Scoping involves defining and understanding the behaviour that the social market practitioner wants to change and how they intend bringing that change about. This is commonly undertaken using *customer orientation* – a marketing term for understanding people's lives such as their characteristics, their needs and desires. This information might be gleaned from a range of different research analyses such as combining publically available data with commercial sector sources. Key to a social marketing approach is *audience segmentation*. This identifies who exactly is being targeted along with their personal characteristics (such as demographic and geo-demographic variables), previous behaviour, and the benefits sought (why people do as they do and what motivates them). Audience segmentation is important because it identifies exactly whom the social marketer is trying to influence, just as in commercial marketing, where specific products are marketed in different ways to different audiences. Finally, in scoping, the costs and the benefits to the target audience need to be understood. This will be related to what people value, and might not be related to health or disease avoidance. As such, social marketing is seen as a consumer-led approach: one focuses on what the consumer needs, rather than persuading them that they need a particular 'product'.

 Activity 9.4

A social marketing intervention undertaken by the US Department of Children and Family Services (DCFS, 2009) suggested that young people would gain respect if they used condoms during sexual intercourse. Consider the benefits that might be highlighted in such an intervention. What might be the costs of undertaking the behaviour promoted in the intervention for the individual targeted by the intervention?

Feedback

In this instance, the individual is encouraged to use condoms so that they can reap the benefits of self-respect and respect from their peers at the cost of using a condom. The costs for the individual might include the loss of sensation or intimacy; the interruption of intercourse to put on the condom; or the cost of purchasing or obtaining the condom. The sense of self-respect and peer respect outweighs the costs of not using condoms.

Development involves establishing what action will be taken to address the motivation (and therefore the behaviour) of the target audience that has been scoped in the first stage. This should involve drawing on theories of change that demonstrate how motivations can be changed, or building on evidence of the success of other interventions. Although many previous social marketing interventions have relied on mass media, social marketing involves more than using mass media to disseminate messages. In fact, good social marketing draws on a range of methods. At this stage of development, consideration should be given to *competition*: what other issues are competing for the attention and time of the target audience. This competition might come from peers or immediate family members who might influence the audience's behaviour, or it might come from wider influences such as organizations or individuals seeking to maintain existing (unhealthy) behaviour. For example, a social marketing intervention seeking to increase healthy diets might be competing with a multi-million advertising campaign for sugary beverages. At this stage, attention is given to the first two of the 4Ps described in Box 9.1: the product and the price.

Box 9.1 The 4Ps of marketing

Traditional marketing takes into account the '4Ps' that offer the ideal marketing mix. These are: product, price, place, and promotion.

- The *product* is not necessarily a physical offering but can be a product (a mosquito net), a service (an eye examination), a practice (hand washing) or something more intangible (self-belief, respect, control).

- The price indicates the cost that the target audience would have to expend to gain from the product. Price might not be monetary – psychological, emotional, social or other costs could be involved.
- The place identifies the setting in which the product will be encountered. This might be a physical place, if the product is a physical offering or a service, or it could be a media setting such as a website or magazine.
- Promotion is the way of producing and developing demand for the product. Given the propensity of social marketing to use mass media, promotion is often mistakenly seen as the totality of social marketing. Rather, it is the vehicle by which the product is promoted.

These 4Ps combined are known as the marketing mix, with each working together to ensure that the customer's needs are best met.

After development comes implementation. *Implementation* involves the delivery of the social marketing intervention. This is the most visible stage of the intervention. At this stage, attention is given to the latter two of the 4Ps described in Box 9.1: place and promotion.

The penultimate stage of *evaluation* explores if the social marketing met its stated aims and reached the target audience, if it brought about the desired behaviour change, and if there were any unintended outcomes as a result of undertaking the intervention. As Chapter 4 explored, a process evaluation might be undertaken throughout the implementation of the intervention to explore what can be learnt from this.

The final stage of *follow-up* reviews the social marketing intervention and identifies the lessons learnt for future interventions. This stage might include exchanging evaluation results with stakeholders and reviewing what might be done differently if the intervention was undertaken again in the future.

Establishing benchmark criteria for social marketing

As social marketing has developed and its use has increased over a wide range of issues, attempts have been made to establish what 'good' social marketing looks like. The National Social Media Centre (2011) has developed benchmark criteria to improve the impact of social marketing interventions. Reviewing successful social marketing interventions and drawing out the common elements that contributed to their success, the Centre developed eight criteria. They aim to support a better understanding of social marketing principles and promote a consistent approach to social marketing interventions and their evaluation. The eight principles are as follows:

1 *Behaviour* – the intervention aims to change people's actual behaviour and not just knowledge, attitudes, and beliefs.
2 *Customer orientation* – the intervention fully understands the audience and how they behave through a mix of data sources and research methods.
3 *Theory* – the intervention uses behavioural theories to inform it.
4 *Insight* – the intervention understands 'actionable insights' of what moves and motivates the audience. This includes emotional as well as physical barriers to changing behaviour.
5 *Exchange* – the intervention considers the benefits and costs of behaviour change and maximizes the benefits.

6 *Competition* – the intervention seeks to identify what is competing for the audience's time and attention and develops ways of minimizing the impact of competition.

7 *Segmentation* – the intervention acknowledges that different groups have different needs and desires, and segments and tailors interventions accordingly.

8 *Methods mix* – the intervention uses a mix of methods to bring about behaviour changes and uses all elements of the 4Ps marketing mix.

The role of social marketing in health promotion

As social marketing approaches to improving health have proliferated, some commentators have questioned the utility of the approach and the extent to which it fits within the ethos of health promotion. If health promotion is, as the Ottawa Charter defines, the process of enabling individuals to take control over their own health, then can an approach that attempts to use persuasion, or that determines what the 'right' behaviours are for specific audiences, be seen as health promotion? In addition, arguments have been made that social marketing relies on motivation to change behaviour, without taking into account that individuals also need power to change behaviours and that social marketing has a limited capacity to tackle social determinants of health. Grier and Bryant (2005) argue that social marketing can be used to influence policy-makers who can address those broader determinants of health, although evidence does not suggest that this occurs with regularity or success.

Evidence on social marketing in health promotion

As with many other approaches, the evidence on social marketing to improve health is mixed. A 2007 systematic review (Stead *et al.*, 2007) of social marketing in practice on substance, alcohol, and tobacco use found that social marketing interventions had a positive impact in the short term but that the effects dissipated over time. The review acknowledged that these effects were broadly similar to those seen in reviews of other types of substance use interventions. A European evidence review of social marketing for the prevention and control of communicable diseases (MacDonald *et al.*, 2012) found evidence of positive impacts of interventions on communicable disease related health, particularly in hand washing and sexual health, but less so in other disease areas. It found there was a lack of conceptual clarity in international and European studies in what constituted social marketing (that is, some interventions that are described as such might not be) and that while many studies described the promotion element of the 4Ps described in Box 9.1, the other elements were less thoroughly described. This supports a critique that some social marketing focuses on and sees the intervention as being about 'promotion' while neglecting product, price, and place. Finally, the review found no evidence of social marketing being applied to disadvantaged or hard-to-reach groups, despite the potential suitability and applicability of the approach to do so.

Summary

This chapter has explored the strengths and the weaknesses of using mass media and has raised questions about the limitations of this popular and widespread method in health promotion. Mass media has the strength of putting issues on the public agenda, of raising consciousness about health issues, and of conveying simple information. It is less effective in conveying complex information, teaching skills, shifting attitudes and beliefs, and changing behaviours without the help of other enabling factors. Mass media has a wider reach than many other face-to-face health promotion methods and is an important source of health information that can be directed to and support more complex health promotion methods.

The advent of social media and the technologies that accompany it have democratized health promotion methods. The proliferation of social media provides opportunities to engage with new audiences and to develop interventions that rely on engagement with the target audience. However, there is insufficient evidence about how social media might be used to improve public health.

Borrowing principles from traditional marketing, social marketing has been developed and adapted as an approach to improve health. Benchmark criteria have been established to guide the development of social marketing interventions. Questions have been raised about both the ethics and the utility of using an approach to 'sell' health to a consumer. Although not an approach that simply uses media methods, many social marketing interventions draw heavily on mass media as either the 'product' being offered or for the 'promotion' of that product.

References

Albrecht, T.L. (1996) Defining social marketing: 25 years later, *Social Marketing Quarterly*, 3 (3/4): 21–3.

Bekalu, M.A. and Eggermont, S. (2013) Media use and HIV/AIDS knowledge: a knowledge gap perspective, *Health Promotion International* (DOI: 10.1093/heapro/dat030).

Bryon, P., Albury, K. and Evans, C. (2013) It would be weird to have that on Facebook: young people's use of social media and the risk of sharing sexual health information, *Reproductive Health Matters*, 21 (41): 35–44.

Chou, W-Y.S., Prestin, A., Lyons, C. and Wen, K-Y. (2012) Web 2.0 for Health Promotion: reviewing the current evidence, *American Journal of Public Health*, 103 (1): e9–18.

Collins, R.L., Martino, S.C. and Shaw, R. (2010) *Influence of New Social Media on Adolescent Health, Evidence and Opportunities*. Working Paper. Washington, DC: US Department of Health and Human Services.

Department of Children and Family Services (DCFS) (2009) *Want Respect – Use a Condom* [http://www.youtube.com/watch?v=Grp2ppsigo; accessed 11 September 2014].

Finnegan, J.R., Jr. and Viswanath, K. (1997) Communication theory and health behavior change, in K. Glanz, F.M. Lewis and B.K. Rimer (eds.) *Health Behavior and Health Education* (2nd edn.). San Francisco, CA: Jossey-Bass.

French, R., Bonell, C., Wellings, K. and Weatherburn, P. (2014) An exploratory review of HIV prevention mass media campaigns targeting men who have sex with men, *BMC Public Health*, 14: 616.

Gold, J., Pedrana, A.E., Sacks-Davis, R., Hellard, M.E., Chang, S., Howard, S. *et al.* (2011) A systematic examination of the use of online social networking sites for sexual health promotion, *BMC Public Health*, 11: 583.

Gold, J., Pedrana, A.E., Stoove, M.A., Chang, S., Howard, S., Asselin, J. *et al.* (2012) Developing health promotion interventions on social networking sites: recommendations from the FaceSpace Project, *Journal of Medical Internet Research*, 14 (1): e30.

Green, J. and Tones, K. (2010) Mass communication, in *Health Promotion: Planning and Strategies* (pp. 356–97). London: Sage.

Grier, S. and Bryant, C.A. (2005) Social marketing in public health, *Annual Review of Public Health*, 26: 319–39.

Korda, H. and Itani, Z. (2013) Harnessing social media for health promotion and behaviour change, *Health Promotion Practice*, 14 (1): 15–23.

Kotler, P. and Zaltman, G. (1971) Social marketing: an approach to planned social change, *Journal of Marketing*, 35: 3–12.

MacDonald, L., Cairns, G., Angus, K. and Stead, M. (2012) *Evidence Review: Social Marketing for the Prevention and Control of Communicable Disease*. Stockholm: ECDC.

National Social Marketing Centre (NSMC) (2011) *The Big Pocket Guide* [http://www.thensmc.com/sites/default/files/Big_pocket_guide_2011.pdf; accessed 11 September 2014].

Stead, M., Gordon, R., Angus, K. and McDermott, L. (2007) A systematic review of social marketing effectiveness, *Health Education*, 107 (2): 126–91.

Wellings, K. and Macdowall, W. (2000) Evaluating mass media approaches, in Y. Coombes and M. Thorogood (eds.) *Evaluation of Health Promotion* (2nd edn.). Oxford: Oxford University Press.

Peer education

Simon Forrest

Overview

In this chapter, you will learn about how peer education is used as a method of health promotion. You will explore the key features of peer education and some of the theories about health-related behaviour and peer influence on which it draws. You will be presented with information about the findings of research into the effects and effectiveness of peer education. You will also consider some of the challenges faced by policy-makers and practitioners in planning and implementing peer education and learn about the opportunities presented by social media.

Learning objectives

After reading this chapter, you will be able to:

- describe the key features of peer education
- describe the evidence base for using peer education in health promotion
- understand how to use peer education effectively in health promotion
- describe some of the challenges faced by policy-makers and practitioners in planning and implementing interventions that use peer education

Key terms

Hard to reach: A term used by service providers and other agencies to describe groups who experience social marginalization and stigmatization coupled with a lack of access to and engagement with health and welfare services.

Peers: People who are similar to one another in terms of their age, educational or social background and experience, behaviour, and/or social role.

Peer education: An approach to health promotion that involves supporting members of a group to promote health among their peers.

Peer influence: The effects of perceptions of what peers think and do on the attitudes, values, knowledge, and behaviour of other people within their peer groups.

Young people: People in the period of transition between childhood and adulthood and therefore generally aged between 12 and 25 years old.

What is peer education?

Peer education is a method that is regularly used in health promotion interventions that involves supporting members of a group to promote health among their peers. Peer education may seek to disseminate information, change attitudes, values, and/or behaviours.

Peer education can therefore be seen as a way of using existing social and peer networks as a means through which health promotion can take place. It derives its power from characteristics assumed to exist in relationships between people in such networks, including trust, rapport, empathy, open and informal communication, shared attitudes and beliefs, and the power of influence. Health promoters seek to use these connections and dynamics to achieve positive changes in people's health by providing information and resources to a target group or population through their intervention with individuals within this group.

It is important to note that despite the widespread use of peer education in health promotion, there is no single, universally agreed definition. For example, all of the following definitions relate to peer education involving young people.

. . . young people teaching other young people . . . (Clements and Buczkiewicz, 1993)

. . . an approach whereby a minority of peer representatives from a group or population actively attempt to inform and influence the majority. (Svenson, 1998)

. . . an approach which empowers young people to work with other young people, and which draws on the positive strength of the peer group. By means of appropriate training and support the young people become active players in the educational process rather than the passive recipients of a set message. (Jacquet et al., 1996)

. . . a process whereby well trained and motivated young people undertake informal or organized educational activities with their peers (those similar to themselves in age, background, or interests). (UNFPA/FHI, 2005)

✎ Activity 10.1

What are the common elements in the four definitions provided above and in what ways do they differ? Why is that the case?

Feedback

You will have noted the variability in the specificity and detail in each definition. You will have thought about the extent to which they describe or imply particular structures or relationships between the people involved – the UNFPA/FHI definition (2005) goes so far as to describe peer educators as 'well trained and motivated'. Some of the reasons for the diversity in definitions of peer education are explored below.

How peer education is used

Peer education is used to address a wide variety of health-related concerns and problems and may target one or more of a wide range of groups or populations. For example, peer education has been widely employed as an approach to targeting people with information about sexual health, especially sexually transmitted infections (STIs) including HIV, contraception, and safer sex. Young people, gay men and other men who have sex with men (MSM), commercial sex workers and their clients, and intravenous drug users (IVDUs) are prominent target groups. Peer education has also been used to try to reduce uptake and promote cessation of smoking among young people, and to reduce or prevent alcohol and substance use. It has been used to promote breastfeeding among mothers and to spread information about prevention of diseases such as rubella.

It is noteworthy that peer education is often used as an approach to target young people with sexual health promotions, including HIV prevention. The focus on young people may reflect assumptions about the ability of the peer group to influence attitudes, beliefs, and behaviour during adolescence. In addition, young people are often perceived to be an important target for health promotion interventions seeking to establish positive behaviours or prevent the onset of risky behaviours. The focus on groups such as gay men, MSM, commercial sex workers, and IVDUs is because they often do not engage with other forms of health promotion or health services and have, therefore, been identified as 'hard to reach' by service providers. A combination of social marginalization and stigmatization together with lack of access to and engagement with health and welfare services means that professionals have had to find non-traditional ways of engaging with and disseminating information to these groups. People in these groups may also have low levels of trust in professionals who represent statutory or formal agencies, as well as concerns about their motives. This may especially be the case where behaviour in the target group is subject to social or political censure or outside the law.

The topical focus on HIV and sexual health promotion in part reflects the urgent demands for intervention posed by the rapid spread of HIV and other STIs from the late 1980s onward, and the fact that the subjects and behaviours that such interventions must address are sensitive and complex. Spreading information through peer networks is seen as a way of breaking down some of the barriers to talking about sensitive issues and promoting risk- or harm-reducing behaviours through role modelling. In some contexts where resources are limited – including human, material, and infrastructural resources – peer education has been perceived to be a relatively low-cost approach to intervention.

 Activity 10.2

Think of a vulnerable, marginalized or 'hard-to-reach' target group for health promotion in your country. Why might peer education be a particularly appealing approach to health promotion for policy-makers and practitioners seeking to target that group?

Feedback

Using the ideas above about peer education being a way of reaching people who are not affected by or do not access other forms of health promotion, you might have come up with the following:

- Peer education is a way for an institution or authority to influence a target group that would otherwise be resistant or reluctant to engage directly with a message-giver.

- There may be ideological or principled reasons for peer education, including believing that health promotion should empower groups and be 'bottom-up' rather than 'top-down'.
- Peer education may also be seen to embody in practice theoretical elements associated with effective health promotion. This concept is explored in more detail later in this chapter.
- Peer education includes some strong assumptions about peer influence within social networks being extensive and effective in tackling behaviours that are otherwise very hard to change.
- In some contexts, peer education may offer a solution to identifying the human resources required for health promotion.

Peer education: history and theory

The reasons why there is no single agreed definition of peer education include the short timeframe and diversity of contexts in which peer review practice has developed. The history and origins of peer education are also unclear. It has been suggested, for example, that peer education has pedagogical roots in a form of tutoring popular in Victorian Britain, in which older pupils were paid by teachers to help them manage large, mixed-age group classrooms by acting as 'monitors' (Cowie, 2011). While this has similarities with some forms of peer education, especially among young people and interventions carried out in formal settings, it does not reflect relationships in other contexts, where peer educators are not situated in the power or age relationships and roles implied by this model. It also does not involve any mobilization of the target group as active players in deciding the content or form of any information or learning that is being transmitted to peers, which is often a component of peer education.

In addition, peer education draws on a variety of learning, peer influence, and psychosocial theories of health-related behaviour. The first group of theories it draws on includes Lev Vygotsky's (1978) work on zones of proximal learning. This theory proposes that changes in knowledge and understanding occur incrementally and are in important ways driven by collaboration with near-peers. Vygotsky suggested that we acquire new knowledge through additive learning, which takes place both physically and metaphorically alongside peers whose levels of knowledge and understanding represent the next step in our own intellectual development. The work of Albert Bandura (1977) on social learning has also been influential for peer education. Bandura places particular emphasis on the part played by role models in influencing learning and behaviour. His theory posits that we learn from observation of others and that we adopt their behaviour because we perceive ourselves to be like them in some way and want the approval that flows from emulation.

The second group of theories peer education has drawn on explain how influence passes through the wider peer or social network. The thinking of Everett Rogers (2003) has been influential in this respect. Rogers' work focuses on how a new idea or behaviour passes through a social network via diffusion. The key concept in Rogers' work for health promoters using peer education is that diffusion requires not just a new idea to emerge (the health promotion message) but also communication channels and a social system through which the message can be diffused. Rogers suggested that in any social system there are some people who are 'early adopters' – those who readily take up new ideas and behaviours – and they drive interest in take-up among the wider network. At some point the new idea or behaviour achieves critical mass when sufficient people have taken it up such that it becomes a new norm.

The third group of theories on which peer education draws brings together some elements of these ideas about learning, diffusion, and social influence in the context of various theories of health-related behaviour. For example, peer education interventions have drawn on the Theory of Reasoned Action (Ajzen and Fishbein, 1980) and Health Belief Model (Glanz et al., 2008) among others. Both of these theories propose an approach to understanding health-related behaviour and behaviour change in which both psychological (intrinsic) and social (external) factors play a part. Peer education draws on the emphasis placed by these theories on the influence of social and group norms and perceptions of the relevance and importance of information to the targeted individual. For example, according to the Theory of Reasoned Action, subjective norms – that is, the influence of people in a person's social network on his or her intentions – are a critical element in predicting behaviour. Both theories also point towards the importance of transmission of information and skills in ways that are accessible and understandable to the target group, again a mainstay assumption associated with peer interactions.

The eclectic nature of the theoretical resources informing peer education are constantly developing, with recent work drawing on ideas and ways of working associated with community mobilization and development approaches (for example, Campbell and Mzaidume, 2001; Jana et al., 2004). Campbell and Mzaidume (2001) succinctly describe a community development approach as having three elements:

1 It seeks to empower a community by placing health-related knowledge in the hands of the people affected by an issue or concern;
2 It creates contexts for new identities and social practices to emerge within that community; and
3 It enables the community to support and empower these new identities and practices.

It should be clear that, regardless of whether they explicitly or implicitly refer to theoretical models, interventions using peer education tend to share a similar set of assumptions about the power of individuals within groups to positively influence their peers. Broadly speaking, we can assert that peer education assumes that members of a target group find it easier to relate to peer educators who are essentially very similar to themselves, whom they understand and with whom they may share or have shared their concerns and experiences. It also assumes that peer educators will communicate in ways and forms that are meaningful and intelligible to their peers and that they will provide role models of desired values and actions.

✎ **Activity 10.3**

Imagine that you are a peer educator. How would describe your peer group? If you had to communicate a message about a health-related behaviour, which of your peers would you target and why? In what way would you expect to be able to influence them?

Feedback

Questions you might have considered include:

- Who are your peer groups? You probably realize that you have more than one peer group and you may do different things with each of these groups and act in different ways in their company.
- Did you decide to target delivery of the message to those you thought would be most receptive to the message or to those you thought most in need of it? What influenced your decision?
- Did you take into account your power relationships, such as age, gender, status, and background?
- How did you frame your message in light of these factors?
- Would the message be different for different people?
- What would your motives for doing peer education be?
- Can you understand and describe your approach in terms of the theories described above?

Doing peer education: case studies

To help explore the issue of how theory underpins and informs peer education practice and reflect on impact, effects, and effectiveness, in this section we will look at several case studies of peer education projects.

Case study 10.1: Supporting young people with alcohol problems

The Peer Education Alcohol Project, set up in Scotland in 2009, was funded for an initial period of two years through a grant from a charitable foundation. The project had the following aim: 'to reduce harm and increase access to help for young people who have alcohol problems, increase skills to deliver services targeted at young people and who have alcohol problems, and build closer working relationships between alcohol agencies and young people's services'.

The intervention was informed by evidence from a national survey in Scotland showing that by the age of 15 over a quarter of young people were drinking on a weekly basis and that 43% had been drunk on at least two occasions.

The project recruited 15 young people via a leaflet sent to all schools and community groups in and around the capital city, Edinburgh. The peer educators comprised three young men and 12 young women, of whom 13 described themselves as White Scottish. Recruitment struggled to meet aspirations to attract young people who were perceived to be at serious risk of harm from alcohol use and also from socially excluded backgrounds. Indeed, most of the peer educators had not been drunk, although most had seen a friend inebriated. Their motivations for involvement were to increase their confidence, learn new skills, make new friends, and change other people's lives.

Peer educators were put through an extensive training programme involving training in alcohol awareness and risk-taking behaviour delivered by a national drug and alcohol agency, supplemented with meetings and residential courses aiming to support team-building, enhance knowledge and awareness about alcohol, and develop an alcohol awareness programme for other young people.

The peer-led intervention, comprising structured and unstructured participative activities, was delivered to 232 other young people in small groups averaging 13 members, through 17 sessions in 14 locations (principally schools, youth clubs, and young carers' support groups). The peer educators also devised and delivered two sessions on peer education to youth workers (23 persons) and devised a session for practitioners on alcohol awareness.

The programme was subjected to a multi-component evaluation that included observation of a peer-led intervention, qualitative assessment of outcomes for peer educators, and end-of-session evaluation with the target groups (Lawson, 2011). The evaluation reported a positive impact on peer educators' confidence, happiness, anxiety, quality of family relationships, and attitudes towards school. Pre and post training and intervention measures with peer educators showed increases in their communication skills, empathy, teamwork, and feelings of responsibility. A number of peer educators reported talking to friends about alcohol issues.

Evaluation with young people targeted by the intervention suggested that around a third reported that their attitudes towards drinking had been challenged, and around half had increased knowledge about alcohol issues. Around a third of the target group identified learning about alcohol as the highlight of the session. However, a third did not find the activities enjoyable and a quarter thought transmission of facts the worst part of the intervention.

You can find out more about this project at: http://www.mentoruk.org.uk/2010/03/peer-education-alcohol-project/

Case study 10.2: Peer-to-peer tobacco education and advocacy for people experiencing mental ill health

The CHOICES programme was set up in 2005 to help address tobacco smoking among people registered as outpatients with mental health services in New Jersey in the USA. The project was jointly organized by a university medical school and local mental health service in response to evidence showing the disproportionate number of smokers among people with mental illness, a lack of motivation to quit, together with reduced access to services.

The project sought both to support smokers in quitting and to increase pressure on services to meet their needs by employing peer counsellors who engaged in peer education, outreach, and advocacy. The peer counsellors, who were paid $9600 a year for working 20 hours a week, visited community venues, ran health fairs, and spoke to individuals about their tobacco use. The one-to-one, peer-led intervention took the form of a motivational interview including personalized feedback on a person's health and the social costs of their smoking, as well as information about services that supported smoking cessation. The peer counsellors received 30 hours' training and weekly in-person supervision from a programme director who was an expert in tobacco treatment. The peer counsellors were recruited through job centres and the role was open to any person who had been a mental health service user and who had quit smoking for at least a year.

The programme was subject to an evaluation in 2009 (Williams et al., 2011) which showed that in 5 years, CHOICES reached over 10,000 smokers with mental illness via 298 community visits and met with around 1400 individual smokers. The evaluation was able to assess impact with around 100 individuals. These tended to be middle-aged, unemployed, single people who were long-term smokers. There were roughly equal numbers of men and women.

Key findings were that at follow-up at one and six months, a significant proportion of these smokers had reduced the number of cigarettes smoked, half had tried to quit since the intervention, and 57% had spoken to health care professionals about getting help to quit. The evaluation also showed that peer counsellors reported positive impact from involvement in CHOICES, notably feeling that the work helped their recovery from mental ill health and boosted their self-confidence.

CHOICES produces a newsletter and runs a website (www.njchoices.org).

Case study 10.3: HIV prevention in South Africa – the Rutanang programme in the Western Cape

Following recommendations of the South African Department of Basic Education about components in its strategic plan for combating HIV, the provincial government in the Western Cape has been running a peer education programme since 2006. The programme focuses on students in grade 10 (aged 15–16 years) and has the following specific aims:

- To delay the sexual debut of those young people who have not already become sexually active;
- To increase condom use among those who have already had sex.

The project draws on a broad rationale and understanding of peer education, including a framework and guidelines for peer education in South Africa developed by a wide range of stakeholder groups. In this context, peer education is conceived of as: 'a health promotion and intervention strategy. Peer education programmes target the peer group as the unit of change in order to change social norms and use an individual from the target group (i.e. "peer educator" or "peer facilitator") as the agent of change.' The purpose of peer education is to 'promote the development of knowledge, attitudes, beliefs, and skills that will enable young people to engage in healthy behaviours and improve their reproductive and sexual health outcomes – i.e. prevent unintended pregnancies, STIs and HIV. Facilitated by peers who come from similar backgrounds, HIV prevention peer education programs recognize the important role peers play in influencing young people's behaviour.'

In the Western Cape, the project involved commissioning non-profit organizations at a local level to deliver a programme of peer educator training covering relationships, sexual health and well-being, and confidence-building. Training was ongoing with peer educators offered regular skills training, mentoring, and group sessions every month as well as an intensive three-day training package.

The intervention consisted of a mixture of formal and informal interactions between peer educators and other young people. Peer educators led classroom-based lessons and community-based activities as well as using informal interaction with other young people as a context for information exchange and signposting to services.

The project in the Western Cape has been subject to an evaluation via a non-randomized controlled trial involving 30 schools (15 of which received the intervention). There were no statistically significant differences in impact on the main measures (age at sexual debut, use of condom when last sexually active, and decision-making) between the young people at the schools that did and did not receive peer-led education. There were indications that students in the schools that received the intervention were more likely to start having sex. The evaluators reached two very important conclusions.

First, the effects of social factors such as demography and especially material and social inequalities on sexual attitudes and behaviour are so powerful that the individualized approach implied by peer education cannot overcome them unless they are coupled with community development and initiatives that tackle wider social issues. Among these they draw particular attention to poverty and gender power relations.

Second, the impact of peer education was further limited by lack of fidelity to the programme and structural issues bearing on its implementation. In particular, the organizations tasked with training peer educators often lacked capacity, were not coordinated, and adopted different approaches often influenced by particular belief systems. These limited open discussion by peer educators who, in some cases, were unable to talk about condoms and focused instead on abstinence.

You can find out more about Rutanang at: http://www.cspe.org.za/Peer-Education/rutanang.html

Reflecting on practice

These three case studies show the diversity of interventions that can be categorized as peer education in terms of settings, topics, aims, target groups, intended outcomes, and evaluative opportunities and rigour. They also helpfully illustrate a number of important considerations and issues when it comes to planning and implementing health promotion interventions using peer education.

First, ownership and determination of the 'message' and modes of delivery may vary. In none of the three programmes were the broad aims established by the peer educators but by organizations that instigated the projects. However, peer educators, other actors, and circumstantial factors did influence the message and the way it was shared to different degrees. For example, closer inspection suggests that young people in the Peer Education Alcohol Project in Scotland had quite a lot of freedom in the design and the delivery of the workshops with their peers. In contrast, the content of the intervention in South African schools was not only more heavily structured by the designers but factors such as the views of organizations implementing the training about appropriate sexual behaviour constrained what peer educators could talk about.

Second, there is no single definition of peer. A peer can be defined in terms of age, gender, social status, life experience, and/or health experience. In all three projects, some emphasis was placed on similarity in health status with the intended target group for intervention, be it as a young person who has faced problems associated with alcohol use, a smoker with experience of mental illness or a young person at risk of HIV infection. However, with regard to the Peer Education Alcohol Project in Scotland, information about the profile of peer educators suggests that they did not closely match the groups with which they intervened. The challenges associated with defining 'peer' also relate to the target group. The peer educators in the CHOICES programme made interventions with people previously unknown to them – thereby defining 'peer' primarily in terms of experience rather than as part of a pre-existing shared social network.

Third, capacity to build any social network may be constrained by the nature of the intervention. While the CHOICES programme initiated contact between people who were not initially part of a social network, the nature of the intervention, which focused more on individual peer support than the work in the Western Cape, seems to have the scope to both build advocacy capacity and to lend itself to the creation of peer networks. In this respect, projects of this kind can be seen as generating peer communities. As CHOICES demonstrates, this may be particularly important where individual behaviour change is not perceived to be supported by service provision and where awareness-raising advocacy with professionals is required (Williams *et al.*, 2011: 250).

Fourth, peer educators are beneficiaries of peer education interventions. In all three projects, but particularly the projects in Scotland and the USA, the impact on the peer educators of involvement in the interventions became evident upon their evaluation (Lawson, 2011; Williams *et al.*, 2011). Regardless of the impact of the intervention on the ultimate target groups, peer educators experienced increases in confidence, skills, self-esteem, and personal development.

Fifth, peer education may be project-based and require financial and operational champions. The three case studies reported here reflect much of the practice of peer education in the field, in that they were projects arising from specific and time-limited support from grants or donors and required some form of external leadership to instigate and support their operation. The reliance on short-term funding clearly poses a challenge for the sustainability of a peer education project. It may also mean that a project requires sufficient managerial, administrative, and other forms of infrastructure support to be able to make bids and applications for resources. However, the creation of layers of bureaucracy around peer education may itself be in tension with the ethos of 'bottom-up' and community or group-led activity. In addition, the likely requirement to work to the needs of funders and commissioners can be seen as posing a challenge to maintaining control of the work within the peer education network.

Finally, peer education may be used together with other methods in a health promotion intervention, and interventions using peer education may be part of broader health promotion programmes. The Alcohol Project in Scotland was explicitly situated within a wider programme of policy and practice development. The context for peer education projects may also be set by policy developments as well as infrastructural activity of this kind. In some cases, peer education may be fully integrated into a programme of health promotion. For example, in the UK the APAUSE programme of school-based sex and relationships education includes four one-hour peer-led sessions that focus on the social dimensions of sexual and relational health (Blenkinsop *et al.*, 2004). The aim is to enable young people to explore the motives for deferring their sexual debut, a process in which positive peer influence is seen to play a key part in helping to establish and demonstrate that initiating sexual activity at a young age is not the norm.

Does peer education work? Research evidence on effects and effectiveness

There is a growing body of research that has sought to examine the effects and effectiveness of peer education, with a number of robust studies contributing to the evidence base. One illustration of how far our knowledge and understanding about peer education has progressed is to consider the results of a seminal systematic review of peer-delivered health promotion for young people undertaken in the early 2000s (Harden *et al.*, 2001), and those of a meta-analysis of peer education interventions for HIV prevention in developing countries published in 2009 (Medley *et al.*, 2009).

The review by Harden and colleagues (2001) set out to critically examine the claim that peer education is a more effective and appropriate way of promoting young people's health than other traditional approaches. The review looked at evaluations of 64 interventions that explored both outcomes and process. The majority of the interventions evaluated were carried out in the USA, targeted young people under 16 years, took place in educational settings, and focused on sexual health promotion. In most interventions, peers were either the same age or slightly older. There was a paucity of information about the selection of peer educators but where indicated (in around half of cases) roughly equal proportions were selected by peers and teachers. Harden *et al.* (2001) state that although the vast majority of interventions used peer educators of both sexes, in all cases more females than males were recruited to projects.

The interventions evaluated focused heavily on development of skills in the target group (around two-thirds), with 28% focusing on provision of information. Very few of the interventions were explicitly based on the needs of young people (14%), and in only half did young people have a role in developing or refining the intervention.

Only 12 of the evaluations were sufficiently rigorous to enable the review to assess impact on young people's behaviour. Where evaluation was robust, results were mixed with seven of these 12 interventions judged effective for at least one behavioural outcome, three to be effective for non-behavioural outcomes (knowledge, attitudes or beliefs), and the effectiveness of the remaining two interventions being unclear. The focus of the interventions was diverse, including projects seeking to prevent smoking, promote sexual health, prevent violence, and prevent testicular cancer.

The review included 15 evaluations focused on process, which uncovered a range of important findings. Principally, they pointed towards high levels of acceptability of peer-led interventions. Peer educators tended to be seen as credible, better at understanding young people's concerns than teachers, and making interventions fun, relaxed, and not lecturing. There were some reservations, including that: interventions could be uncomfortable where a peer educator lacked confidence; some young men did not appreciate a focus on feelings; and some emotive topics were not dealt with satisfactorily. Evaluations with peer educators drew attention to the contribution made to their personal development through being part of the intervention, and some tensions around teachers and other professionals undermining the peer educators' control of sessions.

Importantly, research with a similar focus on young people, mainly embracing sexual health promotion, which has taken place since this review, has tended to reinforce and elaborate, rather than contradict, many of Harden and colleagues' findings.

The findings of the review by Harden *et al.* (2001) are complemented and elaborated by those of Medley and colleagues' (2009) meta-analysis. Here the target groups are not limited to young people, and the focus is mainly on resource-poor contexts: places where the impact of HIV is disproportionately high, resources are limited, and evidence about interventions' effectiveness is scant. The analysis focused on 30 studies that reported on interventions in Sub-Saharan Africa, East and South-east Asia, Central Asia, Latin America, and the Caribbean. Commercial sex workers were the target in the largest proportion of interventions covered by the studies (12 of the 30), and young people the target in a further eight. Other target groups included miners, intravenous drug users (IVDUs), prisoners, and transport workers. Outcomes of the meta-analysis showed that peer education interventions had: a moderate but positive impact on HIV knowledge; a significant positive impact on the use of injecting equipment, including reductions in sharing of equipment; a significant positive impact on condom use; and mixed outcomes for STI rates post intervention, with positive changes associated with some interventions offset by increases in STIs in the target population in three studies post intervention.

Critically, the meta-analysis found differences in outcomes between different groups on each of these measures. For example, HIV knowledge was not increased among transport workers, and of the studies evaluating interventions targeting IVDUs, one involving drug users in a rehabilitation centre in China showed no significant impact. Differences by group were also identified for measures of impact on condom use, with the pattern tending towards little or no impact on young people but a significant positive impact on the behaviour of IVDUs, commercial sex workers, and heterosexual adults.

The meta-analysis identified a number of implementation issues that may have been important in mediating impact and outcome. As with Harden et al. (2001), the recruitment of peer educators is identified as important. Across the meta-analysis of Medley et al. (2009), the selection of peer educators varied, with some self-selection, selection by the target group, and by programme or other external professionals. Training and supervision were also identified as important issues. The majority of training for peer educators reported in the studies in this meta-analysis was a one-off training session, the length of which ranged rom a few days to two months. Only five studies reported any ongoing training or supervision of peer educators. Compensation and remuneration was reportedly offered in eight interventions. Retention of peer educators was identified as good in interventions based in schools and moderate to poor in community-based settings and among marginalized groups such as commercial sex workers.

Challenges and opportunities

Despite the growth of both peer education practice and associated evaluative research, a number of challenges remain. Although there is some evidence that using peer education in health promotion interventions can be effective for both knowledge and behavioural outcomes, there are indications that the setting, the target group, and other factors related to an intervention may impact on how effective it is. This requires further exploration.

The relationship of peer education practice and impact to broader socio-cultural and environmental factors is also complex and not sufficiently well understood. For example, there are indications that the ways that power relationships, social status, gender relations and roles, and other cultural and institutionally situated relational dynamics are configured locally and societally impact on implementation and effects. There are particular challenges around recruiting young men to peer-led sex health promotion work and retaining peer educators in marginalized populations and groups.

The diffusional limits of peer education are also not clearly understood. While evaluations often report high levels of target group satisfaction with peer-led interventions, the extent to which messages and indeed behaviours spread beyond the people in immediate contact with peer educators is unclear. And the extent to which peer educators are given or take control of the agenda and the intervention appears limited in some interventions and may call into question the degree to which it is truly a 'bottom-up' approach to health promotion.

While each of these challenges provides an opportunity for development of practice and research, there are also some new horizons to consider. In particular, research on the use of social media as a context for health information and education suggests this new environment has much to offer. A recent review of the literature (Gill *et al.*, 2013) highlights the role played by the internet in both education by professionals and also help and advice seeking by young people in particular (Chou *et al.*, 2009). The internet and perhaps social media in particular are important contexts for the formation of communities built around common interests (Boyd and Ellison, 2007). The scope of the internet and social media as a vehicle for peer education remains under-researched but the potential is clear, as Young *et al.* (2013) found in a randomized controlled trial that demonstrated that peer educators in a US internet network of gay men were able to significantly increase HIV testing and talk about HIV by prompting online discussion.

Summary

Peer education in health promotion involves supporting members of a group or community to promote health among their peers. Peer education may seek to disseminate information, enable the development of skills, and to effect changes in people's attitudes and values. Peer education draws on a variety of theoretical and other resources to explain the ways that it influences health-related knowledge, attitudes, and behaviour. The research base around peer education is rapidly expanding and shows promise in terms of potential for a significant impact on knowledge and behaviour and also high levels of acceptability of the intervention among target groups. However, contextual factors internal to the intervention and concerning the wider socio-cultural context are important influences on practice and may mediate outcomes.

References

Ajzen, I. and Fishbein, M. (1980) *Understanding Attitudes and Predicting Social Behavior*. Englewood Cliffs, NJ: Prentice-Hall.

Bandura, A. (1977) *Social Learning Theory*. Englewood Cliffs, NJ: Prentice-Hall.

Blenkinsop, S., Wade, P., Benton, T., Gnaldi, M. and Schagen, S. (2004) *Evaluation of the APAUSE Sex and Relationships Education Programme*. London: DfES.

Boyd, D.M. and Ellison, N.B. (2007) Social network sites: definition, history and scholarship, *Journal of Computer-Mediated Communication*, 13 (1): 210–30.

Campbell, C. and Mzaidume, Z. (2001) Grassroots participation, peer education and HIV prevention by sex workers in South Africa, *American Journal of Public Health*, 91 (12): 1978–86.

Chou, W.Y., Hunt, Y.M., Beckford, E.B., Moser, R.P. and Hesse, B.W. (2009) Social media use in the United States: implications for health communication, *Journal of Medical Internet Research*, 11 (4): e48.

Clements, I. and Buczkiewicz, M. (1993) *Approaches to Peer-led Health Education: A Guide for Youth Workers*. London: Health Education Authority.

Cowie, E. (2011) *Education: Examining the Evidence* (2nd edn.). London: Routledge.

Gill, H.K., Navikiranjit, G. and Young, S. (2013) Online technologies for health information and education: a literature review, *Journal of Consumer Health on the Internet*, 17 (2): 139–50.

Glanz, K., Rimer, B.K. and Viswanath, K. (2008) *Health Behavior and Health Education: Theory, Research and Practice*. (4th edn.). Chichester: Wiley.

Harden, A., Oakley, A. and Oliver, S. (2001) Peer-delivered health promotion for young people: a systematic review of different study designs, *Health Education Journal*, 60 (4): 339–53.

Jacquet, S., Robertson, N. and Dear, C. (1996) *The Crunch*. Edinburgh: Fast Forward Positive Lifestyle.

Jana, S., Basu, I., Rotheram-Borus, M. and Newman, P. (2004) The Sonagachi Project: a sustainable community intervention program, *AIDS Education and Prevention*, 16 (5): 405–14.

Lawson, G. (2011) *Peer Education Alcohol Project*. Edinburgh: Mentor Scotland [http://www.ias.org.uk/uploads/pdf/Information%20and%20education/Peer-Ed-Alcohol-Project-2011.pdf, accessed 5 May 2014].

Medley, A., Kennedy, C., O'Reilly, K. and Sweat, M. (2009) Effectiveness of peer education interventions for HIV prevention in developing countries: a systematic review and meta-analysis, *AIDS Education and Prevention*, 21(3): 181–206.

Rogers, E.M. (2003) *Diffusion of Innovations* (5th edn.). New York: Free Press.

Svenson, G. (1998) *European Guidelines for Youth AIDS Peer Education*. Lund, Sweden: University of Lund.

United Nations Population Fund and Family Health International (UNFPA/FHI) (2005) *Training of Trainers Manual: Youth Peer Education Toolkit*. New York and Arlington, VA: UNFPA/FHI.

Vygotsky, L.S. (1978) *Mind in Society: The Development of Higher Psychological Processes*. Cambridge, MA: Harvard University Press.

Williams, J.M., Ganhdi, K.K. and Molnar, M. (2011) Evaluation of CHOICES program of peer-to-peer tobacco education and advocacy, *Journal of Community Mental Health*, 47: 243–51.

Young, S.D., Cumberland, W.G., Lee, S.-J., Jaganath, D., Szekeres, G. and Coates, T. (2013) Social networking technologies as an emerging tool for HIV prevention: a cluster randomized trial, *Annals of Internal Medicine*, 159: 318–24.

Further reading

Swartz, S., van der Heijden, I., Runciman, T., Makoae, M., Rozani, A., Dube, N. *et al.* (2010) *'Think for Yourself – Think for Tomorrow': Exploring the Impact of Peer-led HIV Intervention and Psychosocial Support Groups for Vulnerable Youth in South Africa*. Cape Town: Human Sciences Research Council.

Therapeutic change methods

Lucy Lee

11

Overview

This chapter explains how therapeutic change methods are used in health promotion practice. It discusses some of the main therapeutic approaches to behaviour change in individuals, explores the theories and guiding frameworks used to inform their implementation, and outlines the strengths and weaknesses of these approaches. The chapter then examines some of the factors that need to be considered when designing health promotion interventions using therapeutic change methods. Case studies are used to illustrate how therapeutic change methods may be applied to specific health behaviours.

Learning objectives

After reading this chapter, you will be able to:

- explain the key characteristics of the therapeutic change methods used most frequently in health promotion
- understand the theories that support these therapeutic change methods
- understand how therapeutic change can be used in health promotion
- describe the strengths and limitations of therapeutic change

Key terms

Ambivalence: A conflict between two courses of action each of which has perceived costs and benefits associated with it. The exploration and resolution of ambivalence is a key feature in motivational interviewing.

Cognition: Thought processes that include attention, concentration, perception, thinking, learning, memory, beliefs, expectations, and assumptions.

Cognitive behavioural therapy: A therapeutic change method addressing dysfunctional thoughts or cognitive processes and maladaptive behaviours.

Motivation: Incentives or driving forces that encourage action, in this instance the adoption of health-promoting behaviours or lifestyles.

Motivational interviewing: A client-centred, directive method for enhancing intrinsic motivation to change by exploring and resolving ambivalence.

> **Transtheoretical model**: Developed to describe and explain the different stages in behaviour change. The model is based on the premise that behaviour change is a process, not an event, and that individuals have different levels of motivation or readiness to change.

What are therapeutic change methods?

Therapeutic change is concerned with positive psychological and behaviour change, brought about by entering into a therapeutic relationship at an individual or group level. Therapeutic change methods often used in health promotion include cognitive behavioural therapy, motivational interviewing, brief interventions, and harm reduction. These may be delivered through a structured in-person approach, or self-delivered in a modular or manualized form through books or, increasingly, delivered online.

Although this chapter will focus on the use of methods such as cognitive behavioural therapy, motivational interviewing, and brief interventions, it does not assume that these approaches are preferable to other psychotherapeutic approaches. It is important to acknowledge that therapeutic change methods have been criticized for focusing strongly on adapting and correcting patterns of thinking while neglecting the benefits of deep analysis of a patient's history and root causes of thoughts and behaviours. Despite these criticisms, these methods are gaining increasing traction not least due to the benefits they offer over the common side effects of many pharmacological treatments currently available, and the efficiencies of these methods compared with other psychotherapeutic approaches.

In order to understand how therapeutic change methods work, it is important first to consider the theoretical models that underpin them.

The cognitive behaviour model

As the name suggests, the cognitive behaviour model combines two concepts: cognition and behaviour. Integrated cognitive behavioural models are rooted in the concept that an individual's *cognitions* (or thoughts) play a key role in determining how *behaviours* develop and are maintained. This integrated model provides a more compelling framework by which to understand and address these behaviours than pure behavioural or pure cognitive models, which are rarely proposed nowadays to provide explanatory accounts of complex behaviours (Hupp *et al.*, 2008).

The cognitive behaviour model is the outcome of decades of behavioural science research. Several theories determining that behaviour is the product of an interplay of personal, behavioural, and environmental influences shape this approach. These include social cognitive theory, stemming from the work of Albert Bandura (Bandura, 1986) and focusing on an individual's potential ability to achieve mastery over their environment to suit purposes they devise for themselves. Another influential theory is the biopsychosocial model (Engel, 1977), which locates human experience in the biological (physiology, anatomy, biochemistry), psychological (thoughts, feelings, behaviour), and social (relationships, socio-economic status, culture) spheres and identifies risk and protective factors influencing an individual's health at each of these levels. Bandura's work on self-efficacy, which posits that cognitive processes mediate change but that these processes are altered by experience of capability over behaviours (Bandura, 1977), expands on these concepts.

The cognitive behaviour model is informed by this approach (Bandura, 1977), and states that human experience can be broken down into four factors:

- behaviour (situations, events, actions, skills);
- affect (mood, feelings, emotions);
- cognitions (thoughts, attitudes, beliefs, assumptions, memories, expectations);
- physiology (tension, fitness, diet, health status).

Cognitive behavioural interventions are also largely informed by social learning theory (Bandura, 1977), which construes the maintenance of negative behaviours in some way as behaviours learned to cope with adverse events.

Cognitive behavioural therapy (CBT) arose from this model as a therapeutic tool to help relieve people of psychological distress. CBT can be used to designate a package of techniques in which cognitive therapy approaches are used in combination with a set of behavioural strategies. CBT proposes that people become distressed as a consequence of specific behaviours they engage in and, perhaps more importantly, the beliefs they have about those behaviours. Change in a cognitive behavioural sense determines that an individual must change the behaviour they engage in, and how they think about the world and their behaviour. In doing so, they will modify how they feel about themselves and, if the changes in behaviour and cognition are positive and supportive of a healthier lifestyle, in turn that individual will feel better about themselves and have an improved quality of life. The relationship between these key factors is outlined in Figure 11.1.

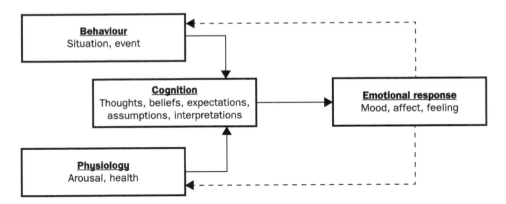

Figure 11.1 A cognitive behavioural model of emotion.

How CBT is used

CBT interventions are designed to address negative behaviours and learning patterns so as to reduce maladaptive or dysfunctional behaviours. They do this through skills-based methodologies drawn from cognitive and behavioural approaches to behaviour change, which in turn draw upon a range of cognitive and behavioural theories such as those described above.

CBT interventions support individuals or groups to identify and understand problems and consider the relationship between their thoughts, feelings, and behaviours in relation to these issues. They focus on current factors maintaining problem behaviours and support individuals or groups to set personalized goals to address those behaviours.

Goals and progress are closely and continuously monitored and evaluated. CBT provides psychological and practical skills to address identified problems, and seeks to provide individuals with the ability to acquire and use these skills. The approach places strong emphasis on setting homework to ensure skills are practised, and puts the control and responsibility for maintaining these techniques in the hands of the individual. The overall aim of CBT is to support the individual – through a therapeutic relationship – to attribute their improvement to their own efforts (Beck et al., 1979; Beck, 1991).

Activities undertaken as part of CBT

The activities CBT involves depend on the psychiatric disorder or problem behaviour being addressed. These can include:

- Monitoring of target behaviour, in an ongoing manner across many weeks, with an emphasis on identifying the situations that appear to trigger the behaviour; the cognitions, emotions, and physiological states associated with those situations; the behaviour the person then engaged in and the subsequent cognitions, emotions, and physiological states achieved as a consequence of engaging in the behaviour.
- Formulations are developed to help explain the relationships between the situational, cognitive, emotional, physiological, and behavioural components in the target behaviour. These formulations can be tested through further monitoring and assessment and can then be modified if required.
- Goal-setting involves setting realistic targets that reduce the harmful outcomes of risk-related behaviour and/or enhance the likelihood of health-seeking behaviour. Graded hierarchies of intermediate goals are then drawn up, so that at any one time the person is only aiming at a target that is slightly higher than what they are already able to achieve, thus making behaviour change more likely.
- Behavioural skills training focuses on people identifying skills that could help them resolve the difficult circumstances previously associated with maladaptive health-related behaviours. For example, the person may benefit from being able to communicate better and being more assertive (firm but polite) in difficult situations, or they may benefit from developing their problem-solving skills, or learn how to relax when feeling physically tense (through progressive muscle relaxation, breathing exercises, walking), or find other more constructive ways of engaging in rewarding or stimulating activities.
- Cognitive restructuring focuses on identifying styles of thinking associated with stressful triggers, including the negative, exaggerated self-talk scripts that do not help the person adapt and cope with an otherwise demanding situation. These can be replaced with more constructive self-talk scripts that help that person focus on the task at hand and direct themselves towards behaviour that helps resolve the situation. In general, this involves replacing 'I can't' scripts with realistic, achievable 'I can' scripts.
- Self-instructional training acknowledges that a person's best behavioural intention can be undermined by particularly acute, demanding situations. Given that high-pressure situations can often be predicted in advance, the person is encouraged to generate a script of self-statements that will help focus their attention on the demands of the adaptive behavioural task (communication skills, relaxation, alternative methods of reward, and so on) that is incompatible with the health risk behaviour. Such scripts help the person stay on task, and can even be used to help the person manage transgressions from their plan, should they occur. Examples include: 'Stop, focus, concentrate'; 'I knew this could happen, so what do I have to do to get through this?'; 'The

tension I am feeling is a cue to begin my coping strategies'; 'Think long-term, don't avoid', and so on. Such a strategy is a key component of any performance enhancement psychology.

- Relapse prevention enables people to implement their intentions to change their behaviour, once they are clearly motivated to do so. It does this through detailed monitoring and identification of the behavioural, cognitive, emotional, and physiological antecedents that precede specific risk behaviour, and the compilation and activation of an alternative behavioural response that can be initiated prior to the risk behaviour occurring.

The ABC model is one of the most commonly used techniques within CBT, aiming to help people analyse their thoughts, behaviours, and emotions. An individual is first asked to consider how a specific thought was triggered (The 'A'; an *Activating event* or *Antecedent*). They then analyse their reaction to that event or behaviour (The 'B'; *'Belief'*). The 'C' is the *consequences* of that behaviour and resulting thoughts, and importantly, the actions taken by that individual in response to those thoughts.

For example, 'A' could be a demanding environmental situation (such as an argument at work or at home); 'B' could be thoughts along the lines of how awful that argument was and how unacceptable it is to have such arguments; and 'C' could be the person engaging in substance use behaviour (alcohol or some other drug). While the consequence behaviour may be the target of concern (substance use), the CBT model argues that the target behaviour will not be influenced successfully until constructive and adaptive changes are made to the antecedent situation (change work or relationship situation, or change the skills with which the person communicates and problem-solves with other people in these situations, and so on), in conjunction with changes in the person's interpretations of such events ('arguments are a normal part of life', and so on).

Evidence of the effectiveness of CBT

CBT has been used to address a range of health conditions. Trials of effectiveness, systematic reviews, and meta-analyses suggest varying degrees of success of the approach dependent on the condition treated (Haby *et al.*, 2006; Lynch *et al.*, 2010; Coull and Morris, 2011). The vast majority of this evidence base comes from high-income countries including the UK, USA, Australia, and Canada. Within these countries, only a limited number of studies have focused on minority populations and most evidence refers to interventions within the general population, accessing primary health care facilities.

CBT has been shown to be effective at treating common mental disorders such as depression and anxiety disorders. In addition, it has been shown to be more effective than drug-based treatment for anxiety disorder. The effectiveness of CBT in the treatment of depression and anxiety disorders provided the basis for its roll out at national level by the UK National Health Service through the Introducing Access to Psychological Treatment (IAPT) programme. The effectiveness of CBT at sustaining improved outcomes for patients after treatment ends provided an additional argument to roll out this programme at scale: the economic benefits created by employment gains and reduced benefit dependency.

CBT has been demonstrated to be effective at improving outcomes for people who experience common mental disorders, but recent research to establish the effectiveness of CBT for severe mental disorders is less promising.

While CBT's effectiveness varies by health condition, the mode of delivery (for example, provider type, training intensity, and duration of treatment) seems to have less influence on patient outcomes. There have been further efforts to explore the potential of adapted models of CBT delivery, such as lay worker-delivered CBT, reduced training duration, and self-guided CBT.

Evidence of the effectiveness of CBT-based guided self-help, including internet-delivered and computerized interventions, is variable and not well established. For example, guided self-help structured CBT seems to be effective at the immediate post treatment stage but less so at later follow-up stages. In the UK, a model combining self-guided CBT with frequent, brief guidance and encouragement from a practitioner acting as a coach is recommended as a low-intensity treatment for depression by the National Institute for Clinical Excellence (NICE, 2009). However, although trials of computerized CBT (CCBT) have suggested that patients recruited through media campaigns (and there-fore self-selected) have better outcomes than those recruited through primary care, CCBT is a relatively recent treatment approach, and therefore the evidence base for its effect-iveness is limited to a small number of studies.

Strengths and limitations of CBT

As described above, one of the strengths of CBT is the extensive evidence base backing the approach for a wide range of conditions, including depression, panic disorder, social phobia, post-traumatic stress disorder (PTSD), and childhood depressive and anxiety disorders. However, while this evidence base provides guidance on delivering CBT within primary care in well-resourced health care settings, and through experienced providers, there is currently less understanding about how effective CBT is in resource-poor settings, or when delivered by non-specialist teams. However, the structured, time-bound, and manualized approach of CBT supports adaptation and testing within new populations and settings. In addition, adaptations of CBT to computerized and online delivery, as well as its potential to be effective when delivered to groups, make it a cost-effective therapeutic approach. Several clinical trials have pointed towards CBT's long-term effectiveness and prevention of relapse (Butler et al., 2006; Hofmann and Smits, 2008).

✎ Activity 11.1

Try and identify the ABCs of a memorable stressful experience that occurred recently. What was the situation (A); what was your interpretation of that event (B); and what happened as a consequence of it (C)?

Feedback

When the links are identified between situations, our thoughts about those situations, and the consequences of those thoughts, it is possible to understand the powerful manner in which our thoughts influence our response.

Motivational interviewing

Motivational interviewing is a cognitive behavioural approach to improving health beha-viours. It is used both as a component within CBT and independently as a technique to tackle specific negative health behaviours and habits, particularly those relating to substance use and addiction.

Motivational interviewing was developed to address problem alcohol use within specialist addiction settings. Rather than using a disease-centred approach that provides a patient with evidence countering an existing health behaviour and justifying a behaviour change to improve health, motivational interviewing encourages patients themselves to identify reasons for and against change. Its focus is on addressing patient ambivalence to behaviour change, employing a series of specific methods to help the patient explore and resolve this through practitioner-guided but patient-determined strategies. The goal of motivational interviewing is to increase the patient's own motivation to change, rather than imposing this on them.

The trans-theoretical model

Motivational interviewing is underpinned by the trans-theoretical or 'stages of change' model. The trans-theoretical model is a temporal framework, determining behaviour change as a process involving progression through six distinct stages characterized as (Prochaska and Velicer, 1997):

1 Pre-contemplation
2 Contemplation
3 Preparation
4 Action
5 Maintenance
6 Termination.

These stages are complemented by processes of change – distilled from analysis of theories of psychotherapy and behaviour change, such as FestingerFe formulation of cognitive dissonance and Bemrm reformulation of self-perception theory (Miller and Rose, 2009) – which identify potential activities to support the development of behaviour change interventions. Implementation of these activities at the correct stage should support individuals to move through these stages. Motivational interviewing interventions acknowledge that people's readiness to change varies, and that interventions should be designed to address the level of readiness an individual has reached to support them to progress effectively towards taking and maintaining improved behaviours. Motivational interviewing is particularly relevant to the earlier stages of change, as it focuses on the identification and resolution of ambivalence about change by asking individuals to assess their current behaviour in contrast to their goals and values. Addressing this ambivalence provides a tool to enhance motivation and initiate and maintain positive changes in behaviour.

How motivational interviewing is used

Motivational interviewing is implemented through a framework developed by Miller and Rollnick (1991). It is underpinned by five principles:

1 Expressing empathy
2 Developing discrepancies
3 Avoiding argumentation
4 Rolling with resistance
5 Supporting self-efficacy.

Motivational interviewing is structured through a phased approach wherein the first phase builds therapeutic rapport and commitment and the second phase facilitates behaviour change through analysis and application of decision-making. Those leading the interviews need to be skilled in facilitating this process through challenging a patient's beliefs while avoiding confrontation. They need to create rapport with the patient, build an understanding of their life context, and put the control for decision-making into their hands. This complexity of approach requires the development of skills over time, and is often backed up with previous training and qualifications in counselling or psychology.

This robust framework for implementation provides structure that supports practitioners in training and delivery, and facilitates planning for service provision. It does, however, rely on practitioners to have an existing level of expertise and requires them to undertake additional training, which, while less intensive than other therapeutic approaches, still poses a constraint to limited practitioner time. In low-resource settings, both these factors make the use of motivational interviewing restrictive, as health workers tend to have limited training – particularly in these skill sets – and less time with patients than would be expected to be committed to developing and facilitating the motivational interviewing process. Adaptations to the motivational interviewing approach address some of these issues, and are described below in more detail.

Brief interventions

As described above, motivational interviewing was originally developed within the drug and alcohol field and implemented by trained counsellors in specialist settings. While motivational interviewing continues to be used for this purpose, over time its approach has been adapted and simplified to address different health behaviours. Much of this adaptation has been driven by restrictions on practitioners' time and this has resulted in shortened alternatives, which can be delivered by less-specialized practitioners and require reduced training time.

One of these approaches, developed specifically to support individuals with a current or potential substance abuse problem, is screening and brief intervention. This approach is designed to motivate those at risk to change their behaviour in relation to substance use. Brief intervention has been developed to treat problematic or risky substance use, but is not intended to treat people with serious substance dependence. It can provide the encouragement to those with more serious dependence to seek and accept more intensive treatment at the primary care level and, if necessary, referral to specialized treatment services.

Brief interventions most commonly take place in primary care settings and range from five minutes of brief advice to 15–30 minutes of brief counselling. The aim of the intervention is to help the patient understand that their substance use is putting them at risk and to encourage them to reduce or give this up. Like motivational interviewing, brief intervention uses the stages of change model as a theoretical framework to guide counselling with patients. The brief intervention is tailored to an individual's 'stage' within this framework, matching intervention approaches to an individual's readiness to change.

The brief intervention most commonly takes place in primary care settings, such as primary care centres, hospital accident and emergency departments, and other community settings. At-risk substance users tend to use these facilities more frequently than the general population, and many common health conditions seen in these settings may be related to substance use. This facilitates a link to providing opportunities for early inter-vention before more severe consequences arise.

One health behaviour commonly addressed by brief intervention is smoking cessa-tion. Consultations with current smokers in primary care can provide an opportunity to support them in reducing or stopping their habit. In the UK, guidance specifies that smokers should receive a brief intervention at least once a year, the intervention lasting for around 5–10 minutes. It involves one or more of the following (Wutzke *et al.*, 2001):

- Simple opportunistic advice to stop;
- An assessment of the patient's commitment to quit;
- An offer of behavioural support or pharmacotherapy;
- Provision of self-help materials or referral to intensive support.

This guidance also recommends that brief intervention for smoking cessation is provided to all smokers coming into contact with primary care and related community and social care services, and places particular emphasis on providing brief intervention to pregnant women and vulnerable groups.

Evidence for the effectiveness of motivational interviewing

There is strong evidence for the effectiveness and cost-effectiveness of motivational interviewing in primary care settings for alcohol and tobacco, although most examples are limited to high-income settings. Motivational interviewing and brief intervention approaches are increasingly being adapted and tested in low- and middle-income settings, and to address health conditions other than alcohol, tobacco, and other substance use. Although the evidence base for the application of motivational interview-ing and brief intervention in these ways is limited, motivational interviewing has been tested in South Africa and Thailand as an approach to HIV prevention in young adults, and has been trialed as an approach to addressing obesity in adults and children in the USA.

Strengths and limitations of motivational interviewing and brief intervention

Like CBT, the evidence base for motivational interviewing and brief intervention is extens-ive and suggests that these approaches can have a positive influence on behaviour change, in particular for alcohol use disorders and smoking cessation. Motivational inter-viewing and brief intervention are less time-intensive than other therapeutic treatment approaches, making them attractive options where services or staff time are limited, and increasing cost-effectiveness compared with other therapeutic approaches.

Some brief intervention approaches have limited success with specific populations. For example, the smoking cessation programme in the UK, which uses brief intervention as a first step to address smoking cessation in primary care, appears to have little influence on pregnant smokers. Additionally, while brief intervention has been recommended as an approach to be used by primary health care providers, even its short duration is seen to be burdensome by many, and the approach is not always followed. In addition to time pressures, the reasons for this may include a lack of tools supporting providers to follow brief intervention guidelines.

A person with a chronic cough is consulting a doctor. The doctor knows the person has smoked for many years and believes the cough is a direct result of the smoking. Consider the following two scenarios and what the smoker's responses might be to each, and which one is more likely to lead to exploration of ambivalence.

(1) The doctor says, 'I know we've discussed this many times before, but we really do need to find a way to get you to stop smoking. Your cough is only going to get much worse and is likely to lead to something much more serious. I can help you to stop, either by prescribing some nicotine replacement therapy or referring you to the smoking cessation nurse. What do you think?'

(2) The doctor says, 'As we've discussed before, I believe your cough is related to your smoking. I wonder on a scale from 0 to 10 how motivated are you right now to stop smoking?' 0 on the scale is not motivated at all and 10 is very motivated. The person gives a score between 0 and 10. The doctor asks why the score is not a lower number and listens to the patient's response. The doctor asks, 'What would have to change for you to give a higher number, feel more motivated?'

Feedback

(1) The doctor hopes to persuade the person to quit smoking by trying to heighten the person's perceived risk of smoking and suggests a course of action. This ignores the person's perspective entirely. If, as is likely, the person feels ambivalent about smoking, they will not only perceive the costs of smoking, but also the personal costs of quitting and the benefits of continuing. The doctor's focus on just one part of the person's ambivalence is likely to focus the person's mind onto other parts of their ambivalence, which they will express verbally. So a typical response might be, 'Yes, but I find smoking is the only way I can cope with the stress in my life.' This type of dialogue will often result in the doctor making the case for change and the smoker making the case for no change.

(2) This strategy is designed immediately to encourage the smoker to express all aspects of their ambivalence without any judgement on the part of the doctor. This type of dialogue will often result in the smoker making the case both for no change and for change, thus allowing them to openly consider their next course of action.

Designing therapeutic change interventions

Most therapeutic change approaches delivered at the individual level rely on the development of a therapeutic relationship between practitioner and patient. However, some therapeutic interventions are delivered to groups of individuals or family members (for example, couples, or parents and their children).

Group CBT is commonly used to address depression, anxiety, and social phobia. Much of the content of CBT focuses on skill-building for the individual and the transfer of techniques for managing problems, and it could be argued that this is no better facilitated by group interaction. The benefits of delivering CBT interventions in groups settings have, however, been identified; for example, groups offer an opportunity to normalize experience through identification with others, and in the case of social phobia, for example, allow individuals to test feared situations such as public speaking in safe environments. There are additional benefits to delivering CBT as group interventions, both in terms of minimizing treatment costs and in improving accessibility to treatment. In the UK, group CBT has been offered on a self-referral basis, and during non-standard working hours, including weekends, supporting individuals who may not address health problems with their GPs to access services with reduced stigmatization.

CBT is also used with couples (to address depression with one partner, or issues with the relationship itself) and families, with particular successes observed in interventions designed to address anxiety disorders in children and adolescents, delivered to both the child and their parents. While CBT can be effective in a group, relational or individual situation, in contrast, adaptation of motivational interviewing to groups is a relatively recent development.

Therapeutic interventions are most commonly delivered in primary care settings. A range of providers are involved in the delivery of therapeutic interventions, including primary care general practitioners, specially trained practitioners, and specialists with defined expertise such as substance use. In some cases, community and social workers are involved in delivery of CBT and motivational interviewing interventions. Increasingly, task-sharing approaches to the delivery of therapeutic interventions are being trialled, particularly in low- and middle-income countries, where delivery of these types of approaches by lay health workers and peers has been tested. There has been a significant increase in self-guided therapeutic approaches in recent years. In addition to guided self-help such as 'bibliotherapy' (the prescription of self-help books to address specific health problems), with the rapid increase in use of, and access to computers and the internet, methods employing online and computerized therapeutic approaches are being tested, refined, and adopted for routine care in a number of countries, including the UK and Australia.

Online delivery of therapeutic change methods

CBT's structured treatment approaches have been successfully adapted to computerized formats. Several systematic reviews and meta-analyses have examined the efficacy and effectiveness of internet-based approaches to prevent and treat mental disorders including anxiety and depression (NICE, 2006a; Kaltenthaler et al., 2008; Lundahl and Burke, 2009; Newman et al., 2011). Internet-delivered computerized CBT (CCBT) has been shown to be effective for a range of mental health conditions in combination with therapist delivery and in fully automated models (Spek et al., 2007). Internet-delivered CBT has advantages over traditional CBT for both client and care system. The anonymity and accessibility of the internet make it very suitable for offering and receiving help with psychological problems. This in turn can reduce the potential stigma incurred by seeing a therapist. There are significant cost-benefits to providing care without reliance on formal facilities, staffing requirements, and compliance with standard office hours. Commonly experienced barriers to care, including accessibility and time constraints, are also addressed through this method. While delivery of therapeutic approaches through computerized methods can remove barriers to accessing care, they are dependent on the individual having, or being able to access, a computer and – where delivery is via online methods – the internet. In more deprived and less resourced settings, this can create restrictions to accessing care. Additionally, while these methods can reduce the amount of time required by health professionals in providing direct support to patients, there is some evidence that some contact with health professionals leads to greater reductions in, for example, substance use. A better understanding of the need for human interaction in health interventions is required to better develop computer-based therapeutic approaches.

✎ Activity 11.3

Computerized CBT (CCBT) is a relatively new approach to delivering therapy to address problems with anxiety, sleeping, and mild depression. There are a number of ways in which CCBT is offered, such as in combination with face-to-face sessions with a therapist and over differing time periods. The scenario below describes a type of CCBT intervention offered within the UK's National Health Service. If this type of intervention was delivered in a different setting, what factors might have an impact on the effectiveness of a fully CCBT course to address depression?

An individual begins to experience feelings of depression and low mood for the first time and after assessment by his doctor is advised to enrol in an online course of CCBT. He follows this course for eight weeks, using his home computer to sign into the website. Although he's encouraged to commit around 50 minutes of his time each week, the course allows him to sign in whenever it suits him, and undertake guided activities and 'homework' designed to make him reflect on his thoughts and behaviours and consider how he might address certain thoughts in a more constructive way. At the end of the eight-week block, he sets future goals and can continue to access all of the exercises he has been introduced to so as to monitor and address his thoughts, moods, and behaviours.

Feedback

In this scenario, the intervention offered to the client was free, and he already had all of the necessary equipment to follow the course at home. A course of CCBT can be expensive to purchase outright (although cheaper than a course of face-to-face CBT) and private access to computers and the internet is still challenging in many parts of the world. CCBT offers flexibility and anonymity, both of which can help to address the stigma associated with accessing support for mental health problems, and difficulties accessing it.

For some people, however, having direct human interaction and a stable routine – as may be offered by face-to-face and group therapy – is important. Having access to a therapist at the outset, at the end of, and at regular points during a course of CCBT can also provide additional support, improve adherence to the treatment, and may support improved outcomes after the treatment has ended. While CCBT may provide benefits in places where there are human resource constraints, reducing human interaction completely may reduce the effectiveness of the treatment. An additional issue may be around the requirement to read through and complete exercises. While the reading age for many of these courses is set at between 10 and 12 years, for low literate audiences, this type of treatment may not be appropriate.

Case studies showing the effective use of therapeutic change interventions for health promotion

---

Case study 11.1: Adaptation of brief intervention using motivational interviewing in new settings: examples of prevention of risky drinking among students at a Brazilian university (Simão *et al.*, 2008)

Binge drinking has been recognized as a significant factor in burden of disease in Brazil, particularly in young people. Heavy alcohol use is linked to violent deaths in the country and this pattern of alcohol use is increasing. Building on reviews of brief interventions for alcohol use which suggest that education and awareness interventions related to alcohol use are not effective at preventing heavy and binge drinking, researchers in Brazil adapted the BASICS (Brief Alcohol Screening and Intervention for College Students) model to address risky drinking in this population. In a randomized control trial, patterns of alcohol use among university students considered at risk and receiving brief intervention were compared with a control arm. The intervention was based on principles of motivational interviewing and the harm reduction approach. BASICS is an alcohol skills training programme that aims to reduce harmful consumption and associated problems in students who drink alcohol. The key elements underlying this approach include: (1) the application of cognitive behavioural self-management strategies (based on the relapse prevention model); (2) the use of motivational enhancement techniques; and (3) the use of harm reduction principles.

In this study, 'at-risk' students receiving the brief interventions showed a significant improvement, in both the amount and frequency of alcohol use as well as harmful consequences of alcohol use compared with the control group.

Case study 11.2: Systematic adaptation of CBT to reduce alcohol use among HIV-infected outpatients in western Kenya (Papas *et al.*, 2010)

The application of CBT in sub-Saharan African therapeutic interventions is limited, but increasing. Successful application of CBT in reducing risky sexual behaviours among HIV positive Zambian couples (Jones *et al.*, 2005) and improving mood among surgical patients in Nigeria (Osinowo *et al.*, 2003) has been demonstrated.

The decision to adapt and use CBT to reduce alcohol use among HIV-infected outpatients in western Kenya was based on strong empirical support for the approach of its effectiveness in both individual and group formats in reducing substance abuse in other settings. Alcohol has been associated with the HIV epidemic in sub-Saharan Africa through risky sex, lowered adherence to anti-retrovirals, and poorer medical outcomes among HIV positive patients. Growing evidence that heavy drinking limits the effectiveness of HIV prevention efforts, along with prevalence estimates of alcohol dependence from several Africa-based studies, led to the development of this intervention to curb the HIV epidemic (Ayisi *et al.*, 2000; Seage *et al.*, 2002).

There are clear benefits to using a CBT-based approach in this context. In low-resource settings, where there are few mental health professionals, interventions to improve mental health may be best addressed through the training or upskilling of non-specialist health workers or others with limited formal health training. CBT holds much promise for adoption in such contexts based on its highly structured format and training approach.

While CBT offers potential benefits related to training, one of the challenges to its implementation in diverse contexts is the need for cultural adaptation to make its therapeutic goals, language, content, and process consistent with those of the target population. Like many evidence-based therapeutic interventions, CBT was developed and tested within non-minority populations in the USA and it was therefore important to adapt it from its standard form to be appropriate to this context. Building an appropriate package of exercises for use with a Kenyan population involved teasing out behaviourally driven concepts of drinking within formative research to ensure that this adapted model was compatible with a local conceptual model of drinking. The package of exercises developed for the intervention reflected the primary focus of CBT – skill-building. Elements including identification of high-risk situations and triggers; examining thoughts, feelings, and consequences related to drinking; problem-solving, identifying risky decisions; and practising refusal of alcohol and other coping skills were included. In order to address myths and misinformation related to alcohol consumption and HIV transmission, methods also included counsellor-facilitated examination of evidence for beliefs, much aligned with cognitive components of CBT.

Case study 11.3: MoodGYM and Psywell

While studies of individually targeted interventions with a primary aim of promoting mental well-being are less common than those delivered at a population level, examples using CBT for promotion of mental health and well-being and prevention of mental ill health are increasing.

Building on the demonstrated effectiveness of CBT in the prevention of depression in adolescents and young adults, MoodGYM is an internet-based CBT intervention serving young people experiencing mild to moderate depression and anxiety, developed by Australian researchers and clinicians (Christensen *et al.*, 2004). There are over 700,000 registered MoodGYM users worldwide. MoodGYM has been adapted to a mental health promotion intervention, and implemented as the 'PsyWell' randomized control trial to promote mental health in the general population in England (Powell *et al.*, 2013). Designed as a fully automated web-based intervention, it consists of five interactive modules teaching cognitive behavioural principles. MoodGYM follows CBT approaches providing guidance on how thoughts and emotions are related, focusing on current experiences and supporting participants to work through common issues such as stress and relationship break-ups. It provides participants with a way to monitor progress, and apply problem-solving, relaxation and meditation techniques in homework exercises such as quizzes.

This is the first trial to evaluate the promotion of mental well-being using an internet-based CBT approach. As such, it holds promise for further application of online forms of CBT to the promotion of mental health in the general population. Participants in the trial's intervention arm achieved significant improvements in well-being scores and self-rated scores of depression and anxiety. It also demonstrates challenges posed by delivery of therapeutic change interventions through online platforms, not least the high rates of attrition found in interventions of this type. Though low rates of adherence are a challenge, this is potentially less of a problem in well-being promotion for the general population than for the treatment of mental illness because it does not raise ethical questions of inadequacy of treatment of a diagnosed health problem. Considering the potential of this method as an effective tool for mental health promotion at the individual level, and the increasing adoption and accessibility of the internet, its refinement and uptake are likely to improve. Indeed, the UK's National Health Service is already engaged in the commissioning of internet-based therapeutic approaches to behaviour change for common mental disorders. These provide online CBT-based modules in guided support for groups as well as individuals, designed to address various health issues, including depression, anxiety, smoking cessation, and weight management. By 2014, access to five providers of online CBT services were being offered in a number of English local authority areas as a part of the UK government's commitment to increasing access to psychological therapies (NICE, 2006b).

Summary

Dysfunctional behaviour in individuals often occurs in response to their desire to avoid or escape distressing situations. Therapeutic approaches to behaviour change provide a range of techniques to address problematic health-related behaviour in individuals that may occur as a result of resorting to avoidant strategies. These approaches tend to be supported and facilitated by a health professional and work by encouraging individuals to identify relationships between their thoughts and behaviours. Individuals are provided with skills and methods to improve their ability to identify and change behaviours. They include cognitive behavioural therapy, motivational interviewing, brief intervention, and adaptations of these models to provide computerized and manualized interventions.

Cognitive behavioural therapy, motivational interviewing, and brief intervention are evidence-based approaches to behaviour change, and provide robust, tested intervention models that hold promise for adaptation to a variety of settings and populations. In addition, a growing number of systematic reviews and meta-analyses suggest that approaches such as CBT and motivational interviewing can be cost-effective to implement for a range of health conditions (Mitte, 2005).

References

Ayisi, J.G., van Eijk, A.M., ter Kuil, F.O., Koiczak, M.S., Otieno, J.A., Misore, A.O. *et al.* (2000) Risk factors for HIV infection among asymptomatic pregnant women attending an antenatal clinic in western Kenya, *International Journal of STD and AIDS*, 11: 393–401.

Bandura, A. (1977) Self-efficacy: toward a unifying theory of behavioural change, *Psychological Review*, 84 (2): 191–215.

Bandura, A. (1986) *Social Foundations of Thought and Action: A Social Cognitive Theory*. Englewood Cliffs, NJ: Prentice-Hall.

Beck, A.T. (1991) Cognitive therapy: a 30-year retrospective, *American Psychologist*, 46 (4): 368–75.

Beck, A.T., Rush, A.J., Shaw, B.F. and Emery, G. (1979) *Cognitive Therapy of Depression*. New York: Guilford Press.

Butler, A.C., Chapman, J.E., Forman, E.M. and Beck, A.T. (2006) The empirical status of cognitive-behavioral therapy: a review of meta-analyses, *Clinical Psychology Review*, 26 (1): 17–31.

Christensen, H., Griffiths, K.M. and Jorm, A.F. (2004) Delivering interventions for depression by using the internet: randomised controlled trial, *British Medical Journal*, 328 (7434): 265.

Coull, G. and Morris, P.G. (2011) The clinical effectiveness of CBT-based guided self-help interventions for anxiety and depressive disorders: a systematic review, *Psychological Medicine*, 41: 2239–52.

Engel, G.L. (1977) The need for a new medical model: a challenge for biomedicine, *Science*, 196: 129–36.

Haby, M.M., Donnelly, M., Corry, J. and Vos, T. (2006) Cognitive behavioural therapy for depression, panic disorder and generalized anxiety disorder: a meta-regression of factors that may predict outcome, *Australian and New Zealand Journal of Psychiatry*, 40: 9–19.

Hofmann, S.G. and Smits, J.A. (2008) Cognitive-behavioral therapy for adult anxiety disorders: a meta-analysis of randomized placebo-controlled trials, *Journal of Clinical Psychiatry*, 69 (4): 621–32.

Hupp, S.D., Reitman, D. and Jewell, J.D. (2008) Cognitive-behavioral theory, in M. Hersen and A.M. Gross (eds.) *Handbook of Clinical Psychology, Vol. 2: Children and Adolescents* (pp. 263–88). Hoboken, NJ: Wiley.

Jones, D.L., Ross, D., Weiss, S.M., Bhat, G. and Chitalu, N. (2005) Influence of partner participation on sexual risk behavior reduction among HIV-positive Zambian women, *Journal of Urban Health*, 82 (3 suppl. 4): iv 92–100.

Kaltenthaler, E., Parry, G., Beverley, C. and Ferriter, M. (2008) Computerised CBT for depression: a systematic review, *British Journal of Psychiatry*, 193: 181–4.

Lundahl, B. and Burke, B.L. (2009) The effectiveness and applicability of motivational interviewing: a practice-friendly review of four meta-analyses, *Journal of Clinical Psychology*, 65: 1232–45.

Lynch, D., Laws, K.R. and McKenna, P.J. (2010) Cognitive behavioural therapy for major psychiatric disorder: does it really work? A meta-analytical review of well-controlled trials, *Psychological Medicine*, 40 (1): 9–24.

Miller, W.R. and Rollnick, S. (1991) *Motivational Interviewing: Preparing People to Change Addictive Behavior*. New York: Guilford Press.

Miller, W.R. and Rose, G.S. (2009) Toward a theory of motivational interviewing, *American Psychologist*, 64 (6): 527–37.

Mitte, K. (2005) Meta-analysis of cognitive-behavioral treatments for generalized anxiety disorder: a comparison with pharmacotherapy, *Psychological Bulletin*, 131 (5): 785–95.

National Institute for Health and Clinical Excellence (NICE) (2006a) *Brief Interventions and Referral for Smoking Cessation in Primary Care and Other Settings*. London: NICE.

National Institute for Health and Clinical Excellence (NICE) (2006b) *Computerised Cognitive Behaviour Therapy for Depression and Anxiety: Review of Technology Appraisal 51*. NICE Technology Appraisal TA97. London: NICE.

National Institute for Health and Clinical Excellence (NICE) (2009) *Depression in Adults: The Treatment and Management of Depression in Adults*. NICE Guidelines CG90. London: NICE.

Newman, M.G., Szkodny, L.E., Llera, S.J. and Przeworski, A. (2011) A review of technology-assisted self-help and minimal contact therapies for drug and alcohol abuse and smoking addiction: is human contact necessary for therapeutic efficacy?, *Clinical Psychology Review*, 31: 178–86.

Osinowo, H.O., Olley, B.O. and Adejumo, A.O. (2003) Evaluation of the effect of cognitive therapy on perioperative anxiety and depression among Nigerian surgical patients, *West African Journal of Medicine*, 22: 338–42.

Papas, R.K., Sidle, J.E., Martino, S., Baliddawa, J.B., Songole, R., Omolo, O.E. *et al.* (2010) Systematic cultural adaptation of cognitive-behavioral therapy to reduce alcohol use among HIV-infected outpatients in western Kenya, *AIDS and Behavior*, 14 (3): 669–78.

Powell, J., Hamborg, T., Stallard, N., Burls, A., McSorley, J., Bennett, K. *et al.* (2013) Effectiveness of a web-based cognitive-behavioral tool to improve mental well-being in the general population: randomized controlled trial, *Journal of Medical Internet Research*, 15 (1): e2.

Prochaska, J.O. and Velicer, W.F. (1997) The transtheoretical model of health behavior change, *American Journal of Health Promotion*, 12 (1): 38–48.

Seage, G.R., Holte, S., Gross, M., Koblin, B., Marmor, M., Mayer, K.H. *et al.* (2002) Case-crossover study of partner and situational factors for unprotected sex, *Journal of Acquired Immune Deficiency Syndrome*, 31: 432–9.

Simão, M.O., Kerr-Corrêa, F., Smaira, S.I., Trinca, L.A., Floripes, T.M., Dalben, I. *et al.* (2008) Prevention of 'risky' drinking among students at a Brazilian university, *Alcohol and Alcoholism*, 43 (4): 470–6.

Spek, V., Cuijpers, P.I.M., Nyklícek, I., Riper, H., Keyzer, J. and Pop, V. (2007) Internet-based cognitive behaviour therapy for symptoms of depression and anxiety: a meta-analysis, *Psychological Medicine*, 37 (3): 319–28.

Wutzke, S.E., Shiell, A., Gomel, M.K. and Conigrave, K.M. (2001) Cost-effectiveness of brief interventions for reducing alcohol consumption, *Social Science and Medicine*, 52 (6): 863–70.

12 Information and advice methods

Will Nutland and Peter Weatherburn

Overview

This chapter examines how interventions that provide advice and information are used in health promotion. It describes four key methods used in these interventions: outreach or detached work; group work; theatre or other performance; and interactive radio and other audio and visual methods. The chapter outlines how these methods are similar and complementary to other health promotion methods, and their distinguishing features. The chapter goes on to provide case studies of example interventions that use information and advice methods, and then outlines the strengths and weaknesses of these methods in practice.

Learning objectives

After reading this chapter, you will be able to:

- explain what information and advice methods are
- understand how information and advice methods complement other health promotion methods
- describe the benefits and the challenges inherent to information and advice methods, compared with other methods
- understand the application of information and advice methods in practice, drawing on examples and case studies

Key terms

Group work: A method that involves the health promoter delivering to and facilitating a group, usually with a shared set of needs or characteristics.

Information and advice methods: Interventions that involve the exchange of information and advice between individuals.

Outreach work: A method of delivering health promotion that involves the health promoter going to a setting where the target group will be encountered, and delivering an intervention within that setting.

Radio and broadcast methods: Health promotion delivered through radio or other broadcast methods such as television or internet streaming.

Theatre and performance methods: Health promotion delivered through performance such as dance, music, puppetry, poetry, and drama.

Introduction

Interventions that provide advice and allow for the exchange of information are common in health promotion practice. These interventions give individuals direct contact with a health professional or a trained peer. They involve engaging individuals in discussion, listening to their needs, experiences and feelings, and offering information and advice, and sometimes referral to other services. Although the contexts in which individuals come into contact with such health promotion activity varies widely, many core principles of information and advice provision remain the same, regardless of the setting.

In this book, information and advice interventions are distinguished from information-based mass media interventions by their interactivity and the exchange of information between individuals. This is different from the flow of information through mass media or other text-based health promotion, such as leaflets or websites, which is generally one-directional.

 Activity 12.1

Drawing on your own academic, professional or personal experience, identify health promotion information and advice interventions that you have recently encountered. Were these interventions that you sought, or were they encountered otherwise? Where did you encounter them?

Feedback

Examples you might have thought of include:

- Encountering an information or advice intervention on a recent visit to a health centre or a family doctor;
- Listening to a radio call-in show with a health theme, or being part of a film or video showing that was followed by a moderated discussion between participants;
- Visiting a health roadshow in a town or city, with volunteers providing information and advice on a topic like diabetes, blood pressure or exercise;
- Advice from a community health worker on breastfeeding, childhood vaccinations or another aspect of being a new parent;
- Attending a group work programme to help quit smoking, or to learn about a new health service;
- Discussion with an outreach worker in a social venue about sexual health or alcohol use;
- Calling a health information telephone line;
- Taking part in a moderated health chat online.

These examples illustrate that information and advice interventions can take many forms and can occur in a broad range of settings. They can be sought out by the target group, they might be encountered by chance, or the provider of the service might directly approach the target group either because of the setting (such as a bar or a club, a faith centre, hospital, or school) or because the target group is also accessing another service (such as visiting a family doctor).

Information and advice: a gateway to other interventions

While information and advice can be actively sought by anyone, either face to face or on the telephone or online, it can also be encountered unexpectedly in a range of community and commercial settings. Health promoters often use short information and advice sessions as a tool to promote and extend the impact of other interventions, such as mass media campaigns. In addition, it can be a way of promoting or making referrals to therapeutic services, or other health interventions. Information and advice interventions are usually easily accessed and can be described as a 'push' intervention, such as where target groups meet for other purposes (for example, outreach during a religious or cultural event), or a 'pull' intervention, where the target group is coming specifically to encounter that intervention (for example, a call made to a specific telephone information line).

Listening in an open, non-judgemental way helps those providing information and advice interventions to get a better sense of the beneficiaries' needs and how to tailor the information and advice that they give. However, the needs of clients usually extend beyond the boundaries of an individual intervention. That is, clients who access health information and advice services may also need information and advice about personal safety, stigma, equality, and freedom from discrimination. This means information and advice providers need to be ready to address other issues and signpost to additional services. For example, information and advice interventions addressing HIV prevention in the UK will likely also address need around provision of information and advice on welfare benefits, immigration, housing, employment, and training.

Different methods used in information and advice interventions

Much health promotion activity focuses on detached or outreach work as a way of giving information and advice. Centre-based services (offered on a drop-in or appointment basis) and helpline services (offered by telephone) are also common ways of providing such interventions. Since the advent of the internet and the increase in social media technology, information and advice interventions are becoming more commonly provided through mobile phone texting, chat-room interventions on the internet, or through real-time video chat technology. Theatre or performance are also used to exchange health information and advice, with members of the target audience engaging with the performers or, in some instances, joining the performance itself (such as in interactive theatre). Interactive media such as radio, which involves an exchange between broadcasters and the target audience, has frequently been used as a medium of information and advice exchange. This is distinguished from the one-directional radio advertising or broadcasting discussed in Chapter 9.

This chapter now discusses each of these information and advice methods in more detail. It is worth stressing that they are not mutually exclusive, and these methods of delivering health promotion are often combined or used in complementary ways. For example, group work is frequently used as part of an outreach intervention.

Outreach or detached work as a method for advice and information interventions

Outreach or detached work is a method of delivering health promotion that involves the health promoter going to a setting where the target group will be encountered, and delivering the service within that setting. This might be a public, private or commercial space. In some instances, the health promoter will refer the target group to other services or interventions (including centre-based services) or chaperone them directly to a service.

In many parts of the world, outreach has its roots in radical social work and social action, with peer-led health promotion being delivered to marginalized groups who are not able or not willing to access more traditional health services. It has commonly been a method of delivering health services to those whose lives or lifestyles are marginalized, including drug users, sexual minorities, sex workers, women seeking contraceptive or reproductive health services, migrants, and those fleeing violence at home or abroad. Increasingly, outreach has been used as a way of attempting to reduce health inequalities by improving access to health services for groups such as rural or geographically remote communities, and encountering groups of people who might not be accessing centre-based services, such as young people or men.

How outreach is delivered has developed and changed over time. From its roots in radical social action, outreach in health promotion has become a mainstream way of delivering health interventions The most recent development has been conducting outreach in virtual settings, such as undertaking 'net reach' – outreach in virtual communities such as chat forums for particular population groups (Mowlabocus and Tooke, 2014).

Strengths and limitations of outreach work

Outreach interventions have both strengths and limitations. The most obvious strength of outreach methods is that they provide services directly in a setting where the target group is encountered – they take the service to those in need who might not otherwise access it. Users do not have to travel to or be motivated to seek a service. A further key strength is that the highly personalized delivery of one-to-one outreach interventions means they can be responsive to users' needs, in ways that are not possible in interventions where information flows one way, such as written interventions. They can provide more depth and interaction than many other forms of commonly used health promotion. An additional strength is that some people report a benefit from encountering outreach interventions, even if they do not directly interact with them. For example, seeing outreach workers in public environments where sex work is being bought and sold may foster a sense of safety among sex workers with regard to crime or violence.

One of the most significant challenges in the provision of advice and information, particularly through outreach or detached work, is the recruitment, training, and retention of people willing to work unsociable hours who also have the communication skills and sufficient health expertise to deliver the intervention. It is not uncommon for outreach workers and volunteers to face difficult working environments, often working with vulnerable people and sometimes undertaking work that is on the fringes of legality (for example, providing advice on termination of pregnancy in countries where abortion is illegal, or on safe injection practices to drug users when this is forbidden).

Outreach interventions are intensive and relatively expensive compared with some other health promotion methods and will not be encountered by as many people as, for example, a mass media intervention. The target group might not present health needs that the intervention is funded to address. This can provide challenges with regard to evaluation and sustainability of outreach services. It can also provide workers with a dilemma – provide the information they are funded to provide or the information and advice that the user needs. Outreach work can have one compelling limitation: the settings it occurs in are often intended for other activities, including socializing, drinking, dancing, undertaking physical exercise, and having sex. The target group may not want to be approached or engage in conversations in such settings: when searching for or having sex, or using drugs or seeking other recreational activities; or in settings where encounters might be considered risky or illegal such as public outdoor spaces.

Activity 12.2

What might be some of the issues associated with delivering an outreach intervention in a setting where the target group is also socializing? What might some of the challenges be for (a) the outreach workers and (b) members of the target group? How might some of the challenges for workers be practically overcome?

Feedback

You might have considered some of the following issues:

- The target group might not want to engage with the outreach workers when they are socializing;
- They might not want to be identified as part of the target group of an intervention;
- They might have concerns about privacy and confidentiality.

Additionally, if the intervention is taking place in a setting where drugs or alcohol are being consumed, there will be ethical issues to consider. For example, can the client consent to individual information being passed on to another service or to provide information that might be used in monitoring or evaluation.

Challenges for outreach workers include those of working unsociable hours and in challenging environments, as mentioned above. Workers might also face challenges around dealing with people who are drunk, or using drugs, or are in a sexual environment. In addition, workers might face challenges pertaining to boundaries, especially if the setting is one that they socialize in when they are not working and if they are peer-educators. These might include:

- encountering people they know;
- finding out information about friends, colleagues, family members, and peers;
- considerations about if and when they can return to the social setting after the work shift has finished.

Measures to help overcome these challenges include workers operating in pairs in order to ensure their own safety and to protect themselves against accusations of misconduct. Agencies often develop procedural and boundary guidelines for outreach workers that aim to maximize the physical safety and comfort of workers while also ensuring a standardized and reliable service. The providers' credibility is paramount to the success of such interventions, and good outreach practice dictates that workers are trained about personal, professional, and social boundaries during work and about contact with clients outside of work.

What evidence supports outreach interventions?

Research has indicated that outreach interventions are often poorly defined and articulated, making it hard to identify outcomes. As the chapter has already discussed, outreach interventions funded to address a particular health outcome might end up addressing a different set of health or social needs, depending on the presenting issues of the target group. Findings from a UK evaluation of London outreach interventions found that some outreach workers were ambiguous about what the outreach was intended to achieve and who was meant to be targeted by it (Bonell *et al.*, 2006).

This evaluation also found that outreach in commercial venues commonly impacted on knowledge of the target group. Impacts beyond an increase in knowledge, such as negotiation skills and reflection on personal behaviour, were most common when the target group experienced longer interventions. The evaluation found that workers needed both the relevant communication skills to engage in-depth with contacts, and the belief that this was the role of their work, rather than providing brief information-based interventions. The research concluded that outreach in commercial venues can reach sufficiently large numbers to have community-wide impact.

Furthermore, the evaluation supported other findings (Flowers *et al.*, 2002) that venue-based outreach can play an important role in maintaining 'background noise' concerning a specific health issue; that it can be an important vehicle for delivering written health promotion materials; and can be a way of referring the target group to more in-depth interventions where there is more likelihood of personal discussion.

A review of evaluations of sexual health outreach interventions found that outreach interventions are more likely to be effective if they are theory based; targeted and tailored to particular groups, rather than general audiences; provide accurate and basic information through clear and unambiguous information; and have a focus on behavioural skills training including self-efficacy (Ellis, 2004).

Case study 12.1: HIV prevention and sexual health

In the late 1990s, the London-based HIV and sexual health organization Terrence Higgins Trust, like many similar non-governmental organizations, provided health information and advice through a telephone helpline. Available seven days a week until late at night, trained volunteers provided information and advice to callers about HIV and sexual health, and made referrals to other services such as HIV testing clinics. On some occasions callers were spurred by specific mass media campaigns, or their call was the result of an intervention with a face-to-face outreach worker who had suggested they call the centre-based helpline for assistance with a specific information need. Information and advice was also provided by letter and, as use of the internet increased, by email.

Over 15 years later, ways of providing information and advice have changed. Although a telephone information line still exists, more tailored approaches to addressing the specific needs of key target groups have been developed, including:

- Young people can send anonymous text messages about sexual health that are responded to by trained peer mentors;
- Men who have sex with men can encounter a virtual outreach worker on online dating websites who can answer their questions about sexual health; and
- Outreach workers can be encountered in social spaces – such as bars, cafes, clubs, markets, commercial venues, and community and cultural venues.

In another recent development, the organization's website for people living with HIV (myhiv.org.uk) can provide online group advice, including peer advice, to people in the website's chat rooms, and trained health advisors are available through live video chat to provide information and advice about living well with HIV – including advice on housing, financial support, and diet and nutrition.

Activity 12.3

Identify the key benefits of offering a variety of different means to deliver information and advice as outlined in case study 12.1 on HIV and sexual health.

Feedback

The benefits of using a variety of different means to deliver information and advice you may have identified include:

- They enable providers to offer information and advice at a wider range of times;
- They offer a variety of ways to engage with services that might be more appropriate to different target groups (for example, someone who does not have English as a first language might find it easier to speak to someone in person rather than by phone);
- Some of the systems for providing information can be encountered in social settings rather than having to be sought out, and can be accessed on-the-move rather than finding a time when a phone call can be made;
- They allow for greater targeting and tailoring of interventions to key target groups;
- Some of them increase confidentiality of the user, such as anonymous texts;
- Many of the methods offer more interaction and exchange, including with peers and with more than one person.

Group work as a method for information and advice interventions

Group information and advice interventions are delivered and facilitated by health promoters to a group, usually with a shared set of needs or characteristics. These interventions might be a stand-alone event, or part of a larger event such as at a conference or a retreat. In some circumstances, the group intervention might be ongoing, such as weekly group events that build on the previous week's intervention, or a number of group interventions across a day or number of days.

Group events may require the organization of formal venues. Smaller informal settings might also be used, such as cultural and community venues, commercial venues or the offices of service providers. In some circumstances, group work can take place as an outreach intervention, encountering people within a setting and asking them to take part in the activity.

Information and advice group work might also be described as a workshop or training event, although there is no broad consensus about the fundamental difference between information and advice group work, workshops, and training. Training interventions may be more substantially devoted to the acquisition of skills rather than knowledge (such as assertiveness training) and workshops can be therapeutic in focus. Preferred language differs substantially, but it is important to note that not all group work is focused on provision of information and advice, and not all information and advice relies on group work as a means of delivery.

Group work can also involve information being imparted in other engaging formats such as through debates and discussions, theatre and performance, or quizzes and games.

Trained health promoters, and often peers, discuss health issues with participants. Participants can also receive advice regarding specific issues, during question and answer sessions, and by discussing the health issues with other participants. Depending on the setting, group facilitators should be able to signpost to relevant services, provide written health resources, and provide one-to-one information and advice where required, or make arrangements to do so at a later time.

Strengths and limitations of group work

A key strength is that group-based interventions help to give a sense that health issues are open for discussion. This can be especially important if the health area is taboo, or if attempts are being made to address stigma during the group work session. Hearing information from trusted experts, and having an opportunity to ask questions and engage can increase motivation to seek other interventions and services. Although the administration, advertising, and delivery of group work events require considerable time, effort and skill, and can be cost-intensive, their unit cost (the cost per person encountering the intervention) can be lower than many other face-to-face interventions because many more people are able to benefit.

There are several challenges inherent in group work as a method for health promotion interventions. First, information-giving on its own does not meet all health promotion needs. In particular, it does not help to address the situation where a person's limited power prevents them from making choices about their health. Secondly, group work stands to re-enforce health inequity, as those with the greatest social skills, confidence, and interest in a topic are the most likely to want to increase their knowledge. This can lead to a pattern where repeat attendees are the ones who fill available spaces, rather than those in greatest need. Carefully considered advertising can help group information and advice interventions to reach those in greatest need. Thirdly, given that self-referral is often the key to group work interventions, participants will have to recognize their information deficits and be sufficiently motivated to address them. This motivation is more likely when the person and the agency providing the intervention are trusted, and also when potential participants are aware of the likely benefits. Finally, given the broad range of needs that might be raised by participants, facilitators will require training and experience in using a variety of communication techniques. Knowledge on its own is not sufficient, as facilitators will need to deliver the intervention in a way that is engaging and non-judgemental, and which recognizes the diverse values and learning preferences of participants.

Case study 12.2: Weekend retreats for transgender people

TransBareAll (TBA) is a UK community-based project that seeks to increase the health and well-being of transgender people. The project facilitates a range of weekend retreats incorporating a series of workshops. Although the retreats have broad themes, the direction of each workshop is driven by participants' needs. Each retreat shares a common purpose, that of providing a space where transgender people (and sometimes their allies) meet together in a facilitated group setting to discuss and explore issues such as body image, intimacy, physical health, and emotional well-being. For some participants, this will be the first time they have met other transgender people, and the workshops provide the opportunity for questions to be asked, advice to be given, and the exchange of peer information and advice between participants.

The sessions are facilitated by experienced group work leaders. The leaders are clear that although the workshops often raise emotional issues, the events are not therapeutic interventions. As such, participants are asked to consider if they are emotionally prepared for the workshops, and are asked to agree to a set of pre-written ground rules.

Activity 12.4

Using case study 12.2 on weekend retreats for transgender people as a guide, what are some of the key issues that should be considered in planning information and advice group work sessions?

Feedback

You might have considered the following issues:

- The physical space used for the retreats needs to provide confidentiality and meet the needs of the target group.
- The skills set of the facilitators will be important, since it is clear that although a workshop might be information and advice based, emotional or interpersonal issues are likely to be encountered and addressed.
- How will access to more specialist support or advice services be provided?
- How will the needs of facilitators to access specialist information, support or referral be met?
- How will people be recruited to the workshops?
- How will you manage boundaries between facilitators and participants? What are the issues around ground rules for the group work and how might these be drawn up in advance as a 'condition' of participation and negotiated between the group members? How will you ensure the workshop meets the needs of the participants?
- Do you need any information about the participants and their skills levels prior to enrolment and does the workshop need to be tailored accordingly?

Theatre and performance as a method for advice and information interventions

Health promotion information and advice can be delivered through a range of performing arts events such as theatre and performance. Theatre and performance can be devised as events in their own right, or they can comprise one element of a larger public gathering or display such as health fairs, celebrations, festivals, cultural, religious or commercial events, or meetings. Carefully structured cultural productions, including those which use dance, art, music, puppetry, poetry, and drama, provide a multi-sensory means through which observers and participants can gain new insights into their existing experience and knowledge about a health issue. In addition to increasing knowledge, performance can encourage people to explore their emotional responses to health issues (including anger, pleasure, happiness, sadness, indifference, fear), while also enabling people to consider the different outcomes of behavioural choices.

Theatre has been widely used in health promotion to provide an active learning environment, including encouraging exploration of social attitudes and modelling positive behaviours. Its live nature lends itself to interpersonal communication that can assist in personalizing health issues for individuals (Glik et al., 2002). In some instances, it has been used to encourage discussions and expose communities to sensitive and often stigmatized health issues (Moyo, 1997).

Strengths and limitations of theatre and performance

Innovative and creative interventions that use a range of performance media can create unique opportunities to encourage people to explore difficult and complex issues. The dynamic and often informal environments that such approaches help to create are likely to engage those who are not drawn to more traditional health promotion interventions such as written information (Blair et al., 1999). Narratives are an important means of conveying meaning. Through the development of an empathetic response, creative cultural events can provide a powerful medium through which individuals can consider their own responses to their health. The use of oral and visual expression improves accessibility for those who have difficulty with spoken language (Blair et al., 1999). Furthermore, the use of modern and traditional art forms can engender an immediate sense of welcome, belonging, and recognition, although targeting must be carefully considered, as regional, generational, linguistic, and religious diversity means that not all interventions will be acceptable to all people.

Well-promoted dramatic performances and video documentaries can be a very direct means of sharing new information, promoting a service, or challenging thinking about a topic.

Creative cultural interventions have the capacity to go beyond raising health awareness, both in terms of the response of the individual and the wider communities they exist within. Where the intention is to reduce health need, planning must incorporate elements that aim to increase participants' knowledge, will and/or power to increase their control over their health. Effective interventions will require health promotion expertise and artistic input. Often, this will require collaboration between these diverse and contrasting disciplines.

Magnet Theatre, a widely used method of health promotion performance to engage and interact with communities, identifies four principles for undertaking health promotion using theatre (PATH, 2007):

1 It should be participatory and interactive. It should not be didactic or about 'talking to' an audience. Rather, it should engage with the audience, facilitate audience participation, and encourage audience members to speak with each other. Performers and audience members should interact to exchange information and ideas both individually and in small groups.
2 It is audience-specific and aims for a repeat audience. Magnet Theatre targets a particular audience and uses appropriate methods to attract them to a theatre site. Encouraging the audience to attend a repeat performance builds a relationship between them and the performers, allowing the theatre intervention to build on the needs of the audience.

3   *It is venue-specific and has a regular schedule.* A fixed venue and schedule encourages regular attendance.
4   *It is a forum for magnifying positive change in attitudes and practice.* The intervention assists audience members in sharing their experiences with the audience, with audience members learning from their peers.

How effective is theatre and performance in health promotion?

There is a need to demonstrate the consistent impact of theatre and performance in health promotion. A number of studies have explored their effectiveness for addressing health knowledge, skills, and practice. Key themes from studies include (Sawney *et al.*, 2003):

- *An innovative learning tool*: evidence supports theatre as an engaging, interesting, and enjoyable method for learning and an effective way of generating discussion about sensitive health issues;
- *Increase knowledge*: evidence concerning the impact of theatre on knowledge levels is equivocal. Some studies have shown that although theatre can increase knowledge, that increase is minimal. Other studies conclude that traditional theatre in education does not impact upon knowledge.
- *Influence attitudes*: there is some evidence to suggest that theatre can positively influence attitudes but there is conflicting evidence about the extent to which this occurs. Some research suggests that involvement in a theatre intervention is more powerful at influencing emotions and feelings than increasing knowledge.
- *Influence behaviour*: little evidence exists on the long-term impact of theatre interventions on behaviour. A small amount of research suggests that *intentions* to change behaviour increase after a theatre intervention, as well as strategies explored during the performance to deal with difficult situations.

In order to be most effective, community theatre needs to be part of a comprehensive strategy that includes exposure to multiple interventions that are linked and reinforced, such as talking interventions with health workers, or information provided through media channels, such as radio or billboards (IYCN, 2011).

Radio and broadcast as a method for advice and information interventions

This chapter now briefly explores radio and broadcast, which are frequently used to deliver information and advice to improve health. Distinct from radio or other broadcast, including advertising, which involve a one-way flow of information from broadcaster to audience as is discussed in Chapter 9, radio or TV programmes that have a distinct health-related theme can facilitate exchange of information and advice between viewers/listeners and broadcasters. As more user-friendly and cheaper technology has been developed, broadcast methods have proliferated, including cable TV channels and audio and visual channels streamed through the internet (such as YouTube). Broadcast interventions might be delivered as a 'feature' as part of an ongoing regular mainstream broadcast show, or as part of a special series, or, in some instances, as ongoing regular programmes with health-related content. Balick (2013) identifies consistent, ongoing programming, at regular times and days as one of the benefits of BBC Radio 1's 'The Surgery with Aled &

Dr Radha' – a weekly radio show in the UK, hosted by health professionals, and featuring regular specialist guests. In addition to providing a health-related feature in each programme, callers can phone, email, text or tweet their questions and concerns and receive on-air information and advice. In such an instance, although the information and advice is tailored directly to the needs of one listener, there exists a dual role of offering advice that can be applied to the thousands of other listeners who may benefit from the caller's information and advice needs.

Radio in particular has been a popular way of broadcasting health information and advice, especially given the global availability and low cost of radios compared with tele-visions or computers. Radio has one notable advantage over television and computers: it is a light, mobile technology that can be easily transported and does not need a mains electricity supply. As such, the Radio Broadcasting for Health guide (DFID, 2004) argues that radio plays an important role in promoting health for economically poorer people and identifies that radio broadcast contributes to public health in three key ways: stimulating community diaolgue and national debate; providing public information and specialized health training; and stimulating positive social and behavioural change, including decreas-ing levels of stigmatization and discrimination.

Summary

This chapter has described four key information and advice methods frequently used in health promotion practice. Information and advice methods are diverse, and are delivered in ways that people might seek out or encounter unexpectedly in their day-to-day lives. They are often interconnected and compliment other forms of health promotion, such as mass media methods, but are distinct in that they involve engagement and interaction between the health promoter and the audience.

References

Balick, A. (2013) The radio as good object: an object relational perspective on the curative and protective factors of a BBC public service broadcast for young people, *Radio Journal: International Studies in Broadcast and Audio Media*, 11: 13–28.

Blair, C., Valadez, J.J. and Falkland, J. (1999) The use of professional theatre for health promotion including HIV/AIDS, *Journal of Development Communication*, 10 (1): 9–15.

Bonell, C., Strange, V., Allen, E. and Barnett-Page, E. (2006) HIV prevention outreach in commercial gay venues in large cities: evaluation findings from London, *Health Education Research*, 21: 452–64.

Department for International Development (DFID) (2004) *Radio Broadcast for Health: A Decision Maker's Guide*. London: DFID.

Ellis, S. (2004) *Prevention of Sexually Transmitted Infections: A Review of Reviews into the Effectiveness of Non-clinical Interventions*. London: Health Development Agency.

Flowers, P., Hart, G.J., Williamson, L.M., Frankis, J.S. and Der, G.J. (2002) Does bar-based peer-led sexual health promotion have a community-level effect amongst gay men in Scotland?, *International Journal of STD and AIDS*, 13: 102–8.

Glik, D., Nowak, G., Valente, T., Saspis, K. and Martin, C. (2002) Youth performing arts entertainment-education for HIV/AIDS prevention and health promotion: practice and research, *Journal of Health Communication*, 7 (1): 39–57.

Infant and Young Child Nutrition Project (IYCN) (2011) *Community Theater for Improved Nutrition: A Guide for Program Managers and Theater Groups*. Washington, DC: USAID.

Mowlabocus, S. and Tooke, B. (2014) *Reaching Out Online: A Report into the Challenges and Benefits of Using Digital and Social Media Platforms for Community Outreach Work.* Brighton: University of Sussex.

Moyo, F.F. (1997) Drama: an appropriate tool in development support communication, *African Media Review*, 11 (1): 92–105.

Program for Appropriate Technology for Health (PATH) (2007) *Magnet Theatre: A Guide for Theatre Troupes.* Nairobi, Kenya: PATH.

Sawney, F., Sykes, S., Keene, M., Swindon, L. and McCormick, G. (2003) *It Opened My Eyes – Using Theatre in Education to Deliver Sex and Relationships Education*. London: Health Development Agency.

Multi-level interventions and programmes in health promotion

13

Liza Cragg, Adam Fletcher and Will Nutland

Overview

Chapter 1 of this book outlined the complexity of health needs, the determinants of health, and behaviours that health promoters are seeking to address. It also discussed the many different stakeholders engaged in health promotion and the complex issues of acceptability and feasibility involved. Chapters 5 to 12 of this book described in detail a wide range of different intervention methods commonly used in health promotion practice around the world. However, it is widely recognized that due to this complexity, no single health promotion intervention method can effectively address major public health problems because such problems require change at multiple levels, including the individual, community, and wider socio-economic levels. Nevertheless, it is possible to combine more than one health promotion intervention method to address the determinants of health *at multiple levels* at the same time. In addition, several different health promotion interventions, each working at different levels to achieve the same overarching aim, are often grouped together to form a programme. Interventions and programmes that address both individual-level determinants, such as knowledge or attitudes, as well as broader social and environmental determinants are known as 'multi-level'. Although many of the intervention methods described in Chapters 5 to 12 are themselves complex in that they involve multiple interactive components, working to achieve change at different levels amplifies the complexity of delivery, including challenges such as acceptability and feasibility. Multi-level interventions and programmes that combine a variety of intervention methods to achieve change at different levels are also more challenging to evaluate. This chapter outlines the theoretical basis and evidence for such multi-level interventions and programmes. It then explores some of the practical challenges involved by presenting real-life case studies from a range of contexts and settings.

Learning objectives

After reading this chapter, you will be able to:

- understand why multi-level interventions and programmes are used in health promotion practice
- provide examples of how different intervention methods are used in combination to address multiple levels of health determinants
- consider the practical challenges in designing, implementing, and evaluating complex, multi-level interventions and programmes and how to address these

Key terms

Complex interventions: A broad term for any social intervention comprising multiple components.

Method: How an intervention will achieve its aim(s), such as through the use of mass media, peer education or community mobilization.

Multi-level interventions: Interventions programmes that seek to address multiple levels of influence on health, such as through mixing individually focused and environmentally focused methods.

Programme: A number of interlinked interventions (or projects) addressing a common health issue or problem (or a target group). See the explanation of terminology in the introduction for more on this.

The theoretical basis for multi-level interventions

One of the most frequently cited taxonomies for understanding the many different levels of influences on our health, known as the 'policy rainbow', was developed by Dahlgren and Whitehead (1991). This 'social model' of health highlights the multiple 'layers' of influences on health, including: individual lifestyles; social and community networks; living and working conditions; and the wider socio-economic, cultural, and environmental circumstances. This model is shown in Figure 13.1.

While this model has been helpful in drawing attention to what actions might be needed to tackle inequalities in health, it has also been criticized for underplaying the extent to which actions across these multiple levels need to be synergistic and coordinated rather than seen in isolation (Moore et al., 2013). The Nuffield Council on Bioethics (2007) also drew attention to multiple 'layers' of influence on health but polarized the options for health promotion interventions between those focused on influencing individuals' choices and behaviour on the one hand, and legislation to prevent or restrict behaviours that are damaging to health, such as smoking bans or taxes to increase alcohol costs, on the other.

The socio-ecological model of health promotion proposed by McLeroy and colleagues (1988) is a theoretical model of the multiple determinants of health that explicitly highlights both the multiple levels for intervention and how these are interconnected and therefore best addressed in combination. Informed by Uri Bronfenbrenner's ecological systems theory (1979, 1986), the socio-ecological model is explicitly based on the notion that our health and behaviour are shaped by a number of synergistic systems and contexts, which cannot be viewed in isolation from one another. This model identifies multiple, interdependent domains of influence at the intrapersonal, interpersonal, institutional, community, and policy levels (see Table 13.1) and supports the design, implementation, and evaluation of health promotion interventions that seek to achieve change at multiple levels (Moore et al., 2011).

Schools are one setting in which this ecological approach has long been used, for example by educating children about health risks and making environmental changes at an institutional level with the aim of supporting health. Case study 13.1 below describes a recent multi-level intervention trialled in Australian high schools. However, multi-level interventions are now gaining currency much more widely, as it is increasingly recognized that the major problems currently being targeted by health promotion, such as obesity, smoking, alcohol use, and HIV, involve complex multifactorial aetiology.

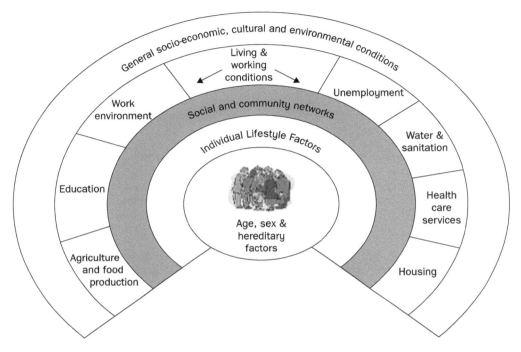

Figure 13.1 The policy rainbow.
Reproduced from Dahlgren and Whitehead (1991) with the permission of the World Health Organization.

The evidence for multi-level interventions

There is strong evidence to support multi-level interventions from systematic reviews, which have consistently found that complex health improvement interventions, addressing both individual and environmental determinants of behaviour, are the most effective (for example, Carson et al., 2011; Greaves et al., 2011; Langford et al., 2014).

Table 13.1 The socio-ecological model of health promotion

Domain of Influence	Definition
Intrapersonal	Characteristics of the individual, such as knowledge, attitudes, behaviour, self-concept, and skills
Interpersonal	Formal and informal social networks and social support systems, such as the family and friendship groups
Institutional	Organizational characteristics and formal/informal rules of social institutions
Community	Relationships between organizations, institutions, and informal networks within defined boundaries
Public policy	International, national, and local laws and policies

Source: Adapted from McLeroy et al. (1988).

Interventions that include higher-level environmental components also tend to be more cost-effective (Chokshi and Farley, 2012) and are less likely to generate inequalities than interventions using individually focused components alone (White *et al.*, 2012; Lorenc *et al.*, 2013).

Many health promotion interventions, therefore, need to address two or more causes simultaneously, ideally targeting factors at multiple levels (for example, individuals, inter-personal, institutional, and community) and comprising multiple synergistic intervention methods. Such multi-level interventions are complex, although their degree of complexity will vary depending on factors such as:

- The number of different methods and their components that are being combined within the intervention or programme;
- The types of outcomes the intervention is seeking to achieve;
- The types of behaviours the intervention is seeking to address;
- The number of groups or organizational levels targeted by the intervention.

 Activity 13.1

Think of an example of a health promotion issue and what shapes this problem. What are the key 'levels' of determinants of this health problem you need to address and which intervention methods would you use to do so?

Feedback

Your answer will of course depend on the health promotion issue you have chosen. However, you should have reflected that any health promotion issue will involve change at more than one level, which will require a combination of different intervention methods. Taking the example of reducing obesity, you may have reflected that:

- At the *individual level*, interventions to improve knowledge, motivation, and decision-making about healthy eating and exercise are required. Interventions providing advice and information, peer support, and therapeutic support may be appropriate.
- At the *organizational level*, interventions need to increase the availability of healthy food and exercise, and change other implicated institutional practices. Interventions using settings-based approaches may be appropriate.
- At the *community or local level*, interventions could work with communities to define and articulate their own needs for healthy environments, including setting up community gardening projects or walking groups or advocating for local traffic calming. These are likely to draw on intervention methods that include community mobilization, advocacy, and healthy public policy.
- At the *national policy level*, interventions such as advocacy and health public policy can be used to secure improvements in the safety of walking or cycling or to improve the labelling of food and drink. Some governments have also tried to use a national 'fat tax' policy to change food purchasing behaviour and improve diet.

Challenges in designing and implementing multi-level interventions

The design and implementation of multi-level interventions and programmes presents particular challenges, including:

- They tend to have many different stakeholders, which can make developing a common vision of what the intervention is trying to achieve and coordinating stakeholders' engagement more difficult. Because of the complexity it may be difficult to ensure that different components of the intervention or programme are delivered in a standardized way, especially if several different organizations are involved in delivery.
- Synergistic components of the intervention or programme are dependent on each other, so if one component falls behind schedule or is not delivered, this will impact on other components and may prevent the intervention achieving the overall aim(s).
- Multi-level interventions and programmes are often designed to take account of specific local contextual factors, so they can be difficult to replicate.
- In practice, they may be difficult to pilot, as they involve the interaction of components that may not lend themselves to rapid testing, such as organizational and policy change.

The length and complexity of the causal chains linking different parts of the intervention or programme mean there can be problems with identifying and attributing outcomes, making evaluation particularly challenging. However, if such interventions are to deliver major public health gains, they must be effective, have sufficient reach, and be feasible to deliver and sustain (Glasgow et al., 2003). This chapter now explores some of the practical considerations that can help support the effective design and implementation of multi-level interventions.

Practical considerations for effective multi-level interventions

Designing and implementing multi-level interventions and programmes requires the same planning and management tasks as those outlined in Section 1 of this book. However, because of the complexity involved in multi-level interventions, several stages require particular attention:

- It is particularly important to explore the evidence base around the proposed intervention, including what evidence exists for each component of the intervention and what evidence exists to support different types of intervention being used together. Ideally a relevant systematic review should be undertaken if one does not already exist.
- It is essential to be clear about what the theory behind the intervention is.
- Testing the feasibility of the intervention by piloting it on a small scale will help identify possible weaknesses. Although it is often not possible to pilot the components of the intervention concerned with achieving change at a policy level, other components of the intervention can usually be piloted.
- Given that several different organizations are likely to be involved in implementing the intervention, it is particularly important to develop a clear management structure with an overall programme manager and clearly defined roles and responsibilities.

- As the components of the intervention are interdependent, it is especially important that effective monitoring procedures are in place to ensure that delays or problems with one component are identified and resolved before they can jeopardize other components.
- Having a project or programme management team that brings together all the organizations and individuals involved in the intervention can help ensure the early identification and resolution of any problems.
- Spending time early on in the development of the intervention to engage stakeholders and to develop a shared understanding of the intervention will help build support.

Figure 13.2 shows a model developed by Craig *et al.* (2008: 8) for the process of developing, implementing, and evaluating a complex intervention. This is also a useful guide for multi-level interventions and it summarizes the main stages and the key functions and activities at each stage. The arrows indicate the main interactions between the phases. Reporting is an important element of each stage in the process.

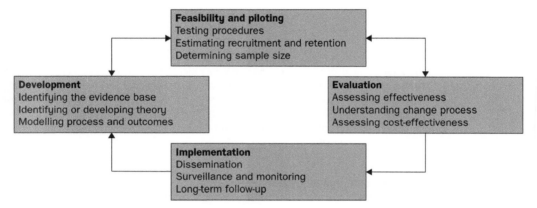

Figure 13.2 Key elements of the development and evaluation process.
Reproduced from Craig *et al.* (2008) with the permission of the Medical Research Council.

Evaluating multi-level interventions

Evaluating multi-level interventions is particularly complicated. Some of the challenges include:

- Understanding the relative contribution of different components of the intervention, and the changes at the various levels they seek to achieve, to the overall outcomes;
- A single primary outcome measure measured before and after the intervention is unlikely to be sufficient to capture the complexity of the intervention's outcomes;
- A lack of effect may reflect problems with the implementation of one part of the intervention or temporary problems in the early phases of the intervention rather than genuine ineffectiveness;
- Understanding the impact of local contextual factors and how changes in these over the lifetime of the intervention affect the intervention's outcomes;

- The long causal chains and time delays between high-level changes (such as policy changes) and changes in individual outcomes.

Thus, the evaluation design will need to be carefully considered. Factors to consider in designing the evaluation include:

- A process as well as an outcome evaluation is needed to understand implementation processes, how any effects of the intervention occurred and for whom;
- A range of primary, secondary, and intermediate outcome measures will be needed to reflect the intervention's engagement at multiple different levels;
- The evaluation should explore unintended consequences through the collection of qualitative process data;
- The evaluation should explore the interaction of the different components of the intervention, including examining whether one or more components of the interventions could have achieved the same results without the others and what was the relative contribution made by intervening at each of the different levels involved;
- The evaluation should describe the impact of local contextual factors, whether the intervention is replicable, and any factors that might affect its replicability;
- The evaluation should integrate an economic evaluation if possible in order to assess cost-effectiveness.

Case studies of multi-level interventions and programmes

The chapter now presents three case studies to explore the practical challenges of designing, implementing, and evaluating multi-level interventions and programmes.

Case study 13.1: The Gatehouse Project, Australia

Informed by attachment theory, which describes the dynamics of long-term human relationships, the Gatehouse Project aimed to improve health outcomes by changing the high-school environment in combination with delivering a new social and emotional learning (SEL) curriculum (Bond et al., 2004). The project lasted for two school years and those schools participating in the intervention began by undertaking student surveys to assess young people's views on local needs and priorities on changing the institutional environment. Institutional action teams were then established in each school, comprising a range of staff and students, to review policies and promote a more positive school environment, which was facilitated by an external 'critical friend' and directly informed by the data from student surveys. The project also included professional training for teachers to support this process of institutional change. At the individual level, the new student SEL curriculum was designed to complement these environmental changes through the direct promotion of social and emotional skills in lessons.

The Gatehouse Project was evaluated in high schools in the state of Victoria, Australia between 1996 and 2001. Evaluated using a cluster randomized controlled trial (RCT) design and compared with schools that carried on with their standard practice, participating in the Gatehouse Project was found to be associated with consistent reductions in composite measures of risky behaviours, including substance use, anti-social behaviours, and risky sexual behaviour (Bond et al., 2004; Patton et al., 2006). Some of the most positive findings were for student substance use outcomes. For example, three years after the start of the project, fewer young people in the intervention group reported having used cannabis in the previous six months and there were non-significant but consistent 3–5% protective risk differences for drinking alcohol in the last month, smoking in the last month, and smoking regularly. The process evaluation also found that the use of multiple different intervention methods functioned synergistically to modify the school's and students' learning (Bond et al., 2001).

It is important to pilot complex interventions before replicating them in other contexts. Informed by the Gatehouse Project in Australia, an exploratory trial of a similar approach to adolescent health improvement through the promotion of a more inclusive school culture was undertaken in English secondary schools (Bonell et al., 2010). This also involved the implementation of a structured 'change process' – involving a student needs-assessment survey, deployment of an expert advisor, establishment of a staff and student 'action team' to review and revise policies and rules using the survey data, as well as staff training to improve communication at school – rather than the delivery of highly standardized intervention activities enforced on all schools. The study was only exploratory, undertaken across four schools, but it clearly indicated the feasibility and acceptability of this flexible, whole-school approach for health promoting change. The results also showed positive short-term effects at nine-month follow-up, as students in intervention schools reported less hurting and teasing of others and were more likely to report feeling safe at school (Bonell et al., 2010). Substance use outcomes suggested intervention benefits but these were not significant due to the lack of statistical power in this small-scale study.

Case study 13.2: Post-exposure prophylaxis following sexual exposure to HIV for men who have sex with men in England

Background and context
HIV post-exposure prophylaxis (PEP) has been used as an emergency HIV prevention treatment within medical settings since the late 1990s, especially in the case of 'needle-stick' injuries. If taken within 72 hours of exposure to HIV, PEP can prevent HIV infection, and is usually taken as a combination of pills, for a period of four weeks. More recently, PEP has also been used for HIV prevention after HIV sexual exposure (PEPSE) in key at-risk communities in many parts of the developed world (Dodds et al., 2006).

In 2003, a coalition of community-based HIV prevention organizations in England, led by the Terrence Higgins Trust, developed an education and policy programme to increase awareness and availability of PEPSE to men who have sex with men (MSM) in England (Weatherburn et al., 2007). Prior to the start of this programme, prescription of PEPSE was seen to be erratic, with MSM having little knowledge about its availability and no official guidelines on if and how it should be prescribed. Anecdotal evidence suggested that PEPSE was being prescribed in a limited, infrequent, and *ad hoc* fashion, especially in large urban centres. Indeed, there was no consensus within the UK HIV sector as to whether PEPSE should become more widely available.

By 2006, the programme resulted in the Chief Medical Officer (CMO) instructing all Primary Care Trusts (PCTs) and Strategic Health Authorities (SHA) in England that the provision of PEPSE should be a key plank of any local HIV prevention provision

(Donaldson, 2006). In 2005 (Hickson *et al.*, 2007) and again in 2007 (Sigma Research, 2008), survey data demonstrated a significant increase in men's knowledge about and access to PEPSE from baseline in 2003 (Reid *et al.*, 2004) across the whole of the UK. By 2010 (EMIS Network, 2013), 54% of men said that they knew about PEPSE; 40% felt confident that they could access it; and almost 5% of UK MSM had received PEPSE.

The key components of the intervention
The coalition used different intervention types in developing this programme and sought to achieve change at different levels. The main activities were:

Building consensus and policy-making
First, before commencing any lobbying or campaigning, the coalition sought to build consensus between key community-based organizations on PEPSE provision. This was important because at such a critical time for lobbying for a change in government health policy, a leading national collaboration did not want to be seen to be pulling in opposing directions. A consensus document was produced that contained key international evidence and frequently asked questions about PEPSE, and setting out the key policy changes that needed to be made to increase PEPSE availability. This document was updated as new evidence emerged and was used as part of a broader influencing strategy to build support for PEPSE (see below). At the same time, coalition members worked with the professional body responsible for sexual health in Britain – BASHH – on the development of PEPSE prescribing policy, published in 2006 (Fisher *et al.*, 2006), and lobbied for the Department of Health's Expert Advisory Group on Aids (EAGA) to publish national policy on PEPSE prescription.

Building evidence
Second, questions about the acceptability of PEPSE and knowledge and use of it were built in to existing community-based MSM surveys, to evidence changes in population knowledge and attitudes over time. Questions about PEPSE were repeated in three England-wide surveys and similar questions were asked in a European-wide survey published in 2013 (EMIS Network, 2013).

Building knowledge through mass media
Third, a pilot mass media intervention was conducted in London and Brighton to increase men's awareness of PEPSE. The mass media work was developed in conjunction with sexual health clinics in those cities and clinics kept data on the numbers of men attending for PEPSE. Once the pilot had been evaluated, the mass media intervention was extended to the whole of England and included targeted adverts in magazines, posters, booklets, and the development of social media. As more MSM became aware of PEPSE, the mass media intervention developed giveaway tools – such as fridge magnets – that men could give to peers with the information: make sure your friends know how to access PEPSE too.

Information and advice
Outreach workers, trained in PEPSE knowledge, enhanced the written information contained in the mass media interventions by engaging with men in clubs, bars, and social venues. They were able to signpost men to PEPSE clinical services or sources of other information and support, as well as being able to distribute PEPSE information booklets directly in to the hands of MSM.

Community advocacy and development
The programme's website developed interactive tools that sought to build community advocacy around access to PEPSE. This included: downloadable letters, explaining what PEPSE was and why it should be available, that PEPSE-seeking men could take to health services (a common issue was that frontline staff, especially at 'out-of-hours' services, did not know about PEPSE); form letters that men could email to the Chief Medical Officer, their local Member of Parliament, or head of their health service, demanding that PEPSE be made available; and a forum where men could post their accounts of having been refused PEPSE (refusals that were followed up by coalition members).

Building organizational capacity
Given that awareness of PEPSE was low in health care settings, and no national guidelines on PEPSE had been published, capacity-building interventions were developed with key health workers. These built on the consensus document and, as well as raising knowledge about PEPSE, sought to allay health professional fears about PEPSE such as services being over-burdened by PEPSE-seeking men.

Media advocacy
Running concurrently with the mass media and capacity-building interventions was a programme of media advocacy. Using the consensus document, and its evidence on PEPSE, coalition members met with community and mainstream media organizations to facilitate media coverage for PEPSE provision. Media advocacy included responding reactively to news stories about PEPSE, as well as facilitating more proactive coverage through articles and letters. Despite one community magazine undermining the evidence base for PEPSE by quoting a doctor as saying it could 'reinforce risky sexual behaviour' (Flynn, 2005), other community media sources played a key role in influencing public health policy: one national community newspaper picked up the campaign to lobby the government for increased provision and covered cases where men had been refused PEPSE. The paper also featured a 'cut out and keep' educational feature on PEPSE that enhanced the mass media intervention that had been run. An unintended outcome of the media advocacy was the threat of a Judicial Review against the Department of Health (Booth, 2006) brought by a man who had been infected with HIV but who had been unaware of PEPSE until the education interventions and the media coverage.

 Activity 13.2

If you were considering replicating the programme described in case study 13.2 in another part of the world, would there be elements you would include or exclude and why? What other methods might you use?

Feedback

- Although we might make assumptions about the relative impact of different elements of such a health promotion programme on its success, it is not always clear if one of the components could have been achieved without the success of another.

- National survey data demonstrated that the target groups' knowledge of and access to PEPSE increased following the implementation of the health promotion programme. It is less clear which specific elements of the programme led to this change.
- While it is likely that PEPSE knowledge would have increased by undertaking just a targeted mass media intervention, it is less clear if PEPSE access would have increased at the same level if prescribing guidelines had not been introduced.
- Similarly, it is unclear if prescribing guidelines would have been produced in such a timely fashion if advocacy interventions had not been employed.
- Although prescription of PEPSE increased, again it is unclear what impact the Chief Medical Officer's instructions to health authorities had on the level of prescribing.
- In addition, it is uncertain to what extent other advocacy interventions, such as encouraging MSM to advocate for PEPSE access, had on PEPSE demand and supply. And were these measures as powerful as a threat of a Judicial Review against the Department of Health?

Your decisions as to what to include and what to exclude would likely involve:

- The resources available to replicate such a programme, including organizational and stakeholder capacity;
- The elements of a programme that are already in place and exist within your setting (for example, if a prescribing policy exists but is not being implemented);
- The capacity of the target group to engage and advocate for change;
- Evidence about the success and transferability of different intervention methods within the programme and the feasibility of delivering them in your chosen setting.

Case study 13.3: The Cardiovascular Health Awareness Program, Ontario, Canada

The Cardiovascular Health Awareness Program (CHAP) is a collaborative, multi-pronged, community-based heart health promotion programme targeted at older adults. It aims to reduce hospital admissions for cardiovascular disease at the population level. The programme, which began in 2000, has been evaluated using a community-level cluster RCT, and includes the following key components:

- Community-wide communication and sensitization ('orientation') with a view to reaching all people in the community who are part of the broad 'target audience' (residents aged 65 years or over), with cardiovascular risk assessment sessions offered free of charge.
- Active engagement of family physicians, nurse practitioners, and pharmacists.
- Regular weekly sessions held in community pharmacies with an appropriate health care professional present, enhanced through explicit links between pharmacists and family physicians.
- Accurate measurement of blood pressure using trained volunteers.
- Referral for follow-up depending on blood pressure and chronic disease risk profile results used according to a CHAP protocol to ensure that participants in CHAP pharmacy sessions are linked to appropriate health providers and resources.

- Global cardiovascular risk factor assessment and education of participants.
- Access to local and provincial/national sources of information and support programmes for modifiable risk factors.
- Feedback of results to primary healthcare provider(s), with participants' consent.

The process evaluation, which was integrated within the RCT of the initiative, found that all 20 intervention communities successfully implemented CHAP (Kaczorowski *et al.*, 2011). After adjustment for hospital admission rates in the year before the intervention, CHAP was associated with a 9% relative reduction or 3.02 fewer annual hospital admissions for cardiovascular disease per 1000 people aged 65 and over. The evaluation concluded a 'collaborative, multi-pronged, community based health promotion and prevention programme targeted at older adults can reduce cardiovascular morbidity at the population level' (Kaczorowski *et al.*, 2011).

 Activity 13.3

Of the different types of intervention you have learnt about in this book, which would you include in a health promotion programme to reduce smoking in your country? What levels would the intervention seek to achieve change at?

Feedback

Reducing harm from tobacco consumption has become an issue of global health concern. Global trade, transnational advertising, and promotion of tobacco products through sponsorship have contributed to increases in tobacco consumption, and the resulting health impacts. Treaties, such at the WHO Framework Convention on Tobacco Control (WHO, 2003), demonstrate the multi-level global, regional, and national protocols and interventions that need to be in place to reduce harm from tobacco (Hawkins and Collin, 2015). These include reducing the supply of tobacco products, and reducing demand for products through both price measures (for example, increasing the cost of cigarettes through taxation) and non-price measures (for example, restrictions on advertising together with education about tobacco harm).

Regional or national interventions have included legislation to regulate and enforce restrictions on the advertising and promotion of tobacco products and sponsorship by tobacco brands. Lobbying and campaigning by health-promoting organizations, such as cancer and asthma charities, have been instrumental in bringing about such restrictions, including the introduction of plain, non-branded packaging of cigarettes.

Increasingly, activities that reduce exposure to tobacco smoke are being introduced and enforced, on a country level or on a state, city or town level. Policies that restrict smoking in workplaces, indoor public spaces, on public or in private transport, or in social settings such as bars, are increasingly common. Central to these policies is an understanding that such restrictions protect workers and the public from 'second-hand' smoke, and that they reduce the opportunities for smokers to smoke.

Further regional or national interventions are likely to include initiatives to reduce access to tobacco products, including restricting sales to minors, restricting settings where cigarettes are available (for example, not close to schools), and reducing direct access to cigarettes within settings where cigarettes are available (for example, under-the-counter in supermarkets rather than in displays).

All of the above involve complex legislative and policy interventions that are frequently hampered and challenged by the tobacco industry, and would need to be initiated and implemented by multi-agency professionals, along with health promoters and public health experts.

However, these legislative and policy interventions need to be accompanied by health promotion interventions at the individual and community levels that support and enhance the more upstream interventions (and are the types of interventions that are more likely to be encountered and delivered by most health promoters). The types of intervention might include: mass media methods that increase awareness of smoking harm, or that direct the target groups to smoking cessation interventions; information and advice interventions that directly target smokers, providing access and referral to smoking services; interactive broadcast interventions that debate and discuss ways of reducing smoking harm; therapeutic interventions that support smokers in quitting or reducing their tobacco intake; settings-based approaches that strive for a whole work-place-based approach to reducing smoking; community mobilization interventions that might seek, for example, to encourage 'smoke-free zones' within a town; peer educa-tion interventions that train members of a target group to provide smoking cessation support to their peers; or advocacy and campaigning for increased action to target sales of illicit tobacco within a neighbourhood.

Summary

This chapter has summarized the theoretical basis for health promotion interventions and programmes that seek to achieve change on multiple levels because there are multiple determinants of health that are interconnected, and these are best addressed in combin-ation rather than seen as polarized or static. There is a growing evidence base that indic-ates the effectiveness and cost-effectiveness of such multi-level interventions. Due to the complexity involved, designing, implementing, and evaluating multi-level health promotion interventions can be particularly challenging. This chapter has proposed some practical steps that can help with these challenges. Finally, by providing case studies, the chapter has demonstrated how multi-level interventions can be used.

References

Bond, L., Glover, S., Godfrey, C., Butler, H. and Patton, G.C. (2001) Building capacity for system-level change in schools: lessons from the Gatehouse Project, *Health Education and Behavior*, 28 (3): 368–83.

Bond, L., Patton, G., Glover, S., Carlin, J.B., Butler, H., Thomas, L. *et al.* (2004) The Gatehouse Project: can a multilevel school intervention affect emotional well-being and health risk behaviours?, *Journal of Epidemiology and Community Health*, 58 (12): 997–1003.

Bonell, C., Sorhaindo, A., Allen, E., Strange, V., Wiggins, M., Fletcher, A. *et al.* (2010) Pilot multi-method trial of a school-ethos intervention to reduce substance use: building hypotheses about upstream pathways to prevention, *Journal of Adolescent Health*, 47 (6): 555–63.

Booth, L. (2006) I realised I had HIV and I didn't need to, *The Guardian*, 23 February [http://www.guardian.co.uk/society/2006/feb/23/health.aids; accessed 5 September 2014].

Bronfenbrenner, U. (1979) *The Ecology of Human Development*. London: Harvard University Press.

Bronfenbrenner, U. (1986) Ecology of the family as a context for human development: research perspectives, *Developmental Psychology*, 22: 723–42.

Carson, K.V., Brinn, M.P., Labiszewski, N.A., Esterman, A.J., Chang, A.B. and Smith, B.J. (2011) Community interventions for preventing smoking in young people, *Cochrane Database of Systematic Reviews*, 7: CD001291.

Chokshi, D.A. and Farley, T.A. (2012) The cost-effectiveness of environmental approaches to disease prevention, *New England Journal of Medicine*, 367 (4): 295–7.

Craig, P., Dieppe, P., Macintyre, S., Michie, S., Nazareth, I. and Petticrew, M. (2008) *Developing and Evaluating Complex Interventions: New Guidance*. London: Medical Research Council.

Dahlgren, G. and Whitehead, M. (1991) *Policies and Strategies to Promote Social Equity in Health*. Stockholm: Institute of Futures Studies.

Dodds, C., Hammond, G., Keogh, P., Hickson, F. and Weatherburn, P. (2006) *PEP Talk – Awareness of, and Access to Post-exposure Prophylaxis among Gay and Bisexual Men in the UK*. London: Sigma Research [http://www.sigmaresearch.org.uk/files/report2006d.pdf; accessed 5 September 2014].

Donaldson, L. (2006) *Improving the prevention and treatment of sexually transmitted infections (STIs) in the UK, including HIV*. Letter to all Chief Executives of Primary Care Trusts and Strategic Health Authorities in England. Ref: 6352, April [http://www.tht.org.uk/binarylibrary/cmospeprecommendations.pdf; accessed 5 September 2014].

EMIS Network (2013) *EMIS 2010: The European-Men-Who-Have-Sex-With-Men Internet Survey: Findings from 38 Countries*. Stockholm: European Centre for Disease Prevention and Control [http://ecdc.europa.eu/en/publications/Publications/EMIS-2010-european-men-who-have-sex-with-men-survey.pdf].

Fisher, M., Benn, P., Evans, B., Pozniak, A., Jones, M., MacLean, S. *et al.* (2006) UK guidelines for the use of post-exposure prophylaxis for HIV following sexual exposure, *International Journal of STD and AIDS*, 17: 81–92.

Flynn, M. (2005) PEP row heats up, *Positive Nation*, 114: August [http://www.positivenation.co.uk/issue114/regulars/news/news114.htm; accessed 5 September 2014].

Glasgow, R.E., Lichtenstein, E. and Marcus, A.C. (2003) Why don't we see more translation of health promotion research to practice? Rethinking the efficacy-to-effectiveness transition, *American Journal of Public Health*, 93 (8): 1261–7.

Greaves, C.J., Sheppard, K.E., Abraham, C., Hardeman, W., Roden, M., Evans, P.H. *et al.* (2011) Systematic review of reviews of intervention components associated with increased effectiveness in dietary and physical activity interventions, *BMC Public Health*, 11: 119.

Hawkins, B. and Collin, J. (2015) Globalization, commercialization, and the tobacco and alcohol sectors, in J. Hanefield (ed.) *Globalization and Health*. Maidenhead: Open University Press.

Hickson, F., Weatherburn. P., Reid, D., Jessup, K. and Hammond, G. (2007) *Consuming Passions – Findings from the United Kingdom Gay Men's Sex Survey 2005*. London: Sigma Research [http://www.sigmaresearch.org.uk/files/report2007c.pdf; accessed 5 September 2014].

Kaczorowski, J., Chambers, L., Dolovich, L., Paterson, M., Karwalajtys, T., Gierman, T. *et al.* (2011) Improving cardiovascular health at population level: 39 community cluster randomised trial of Cardiovascular Health Awareness Program (CHAP), *British Medical Journal*, 342: d442.

Langford, R., Bonell, C., Jones, H.E., Pouliou, T., Murphy, S.M., Waters, E. *et al.* (2014) The WHO Health Promoting School framework for improving the health and well-being of students and their academic achievement, *Cochrane Database of Systematic Reviews*, 4: CD008958.

Lorenc, T., Petticrew, M., Welch, V. and Tugwell, P. (2013) What types of interventions generate inequalities? Evidence from systematic reviews, *Journal of Epidemiology and Community Health*, 67 (2): 190–3.

McLeroy, K.R., Bibeau, D., Steckler, A. and Glanz, K. (1988) An ecological perspective on health promotion programs, *Health Education Quarterly*, 15: 351–77.

Moore, L., de Silva-Sanigorksi, A. and Moore, S.N. (2013) A socio-ecological perspective on behavioural interventions to influence food choice in schools: alternative, complementary or synergistic?, *Public Health Nutrition*, 16 (6): 1000–5.

Moore, S.N., Murphy, S. and Moore, L. (2011) Health improvement, nutritional behaviour and the role of school meals: the usefulness of a socio-ecological perspective to inform policy design, implementation and evaluation, *Critical Public Health*, 21 (4): 441–54.

Nuffield Council on Bioethics (2007) *Public Health: Ethical Issues*. London: Nuffield Council on Bioethics.

Patton, G.C., Bond, L., Carlin, J.B., Thomas, L., Butler, H., Glover, S. *et al.* (2006) Promoting social inclusion in schools: a group-randomized trial of effects on student health risk behavior and well-being, *American Journal of Public Health*, 96 (9): 1582–7.

Reid, D., Weatherburn, P., Hickson, F., Stephens, M. and Hammond, G. (2004) *On the Move: Findings from the United Kingdom Gay Men's Sex Survey 2003*. London: Sigma Research [http://www.sigmaresearch.org.uk/files/report2004g.pdf; accessed 5 September 2014].

Sigma Research (2008) *Country and Regional Data Reports from Vital Statistics 2007*. London: Sigma Research [http://www.sigmaresearch.org.uk/go.php/local/gay; accessed 5 September 2014].

Weatherburn, P., Dodds, C., Branigan, P., Keogh, P., Reid, D., Hickson, F. *et al.* (2007) *Form and Focus: Evaluation of CHAPS National Interventions, 2003 to 2006*. London: Sigma Research [http://www.sigmaresearch.org.uk/files/report2007a.pdf; accessed 5 September 2014].

White, M., Adams, J. and Heywood, P. (2012) How and why do interventions that increase health overall widen inequalities within populations?, in S.J. Babones (ed.) *Social Inequality and Public Health*. Bristol: Policy Press.

World Health Organization (WHO) (2003) *WHO Framework Convention on Tobacco Control*. Geneva: WHO [http://www.who.int/fctc/text_download/en/].

Further reading

Bonell, C., Fletcher, A., Morton, M., Lorenc, T. and Moore, L. (2012) Realist randomised controlled trials: a new approach to evaluating complex public-health interventions, *Social Science and Medicine*, 75 (12): 2299–306.

Chappell, N., Funk, L., Carson, A., MacKenzie, P. and Stanwick, R. (2006) Multilevel community health promotion: how can we make it work?, *Community Development Journal*, 41 (3): 352–66.

Hawe, P., Shiell, A., Riley, T. and Gold, L. (2004) Methods for exploring intervention variation and local context within a cluster randomised community intervention trial, *Journal of Epidemiology and Community Health*, 58: 788–93.

Oude Luttikhuis, H., Baur, L., Jansen, H., Shrewsbury, V.A., O'Malley, C., Stolk, R.P. *et al.* (2009) Interventions for treating obesity in children (Review), *Cochrane Database of Systematic Reviews*, 1: CD001872.

Schensul, J.J. (2009) *Multilevel Intervention with Low Income and Minority Older Adults to Improve Influenza Vaccination Acceptance*. Hartford, CT: Institute for Community Research.

Stead, L.F. and Lancaster, T. (2008) Interventions for preventing tobacco sales to minors, *Cochrane Database of Systematic Reviews*, 1: CD001497.

Glossary

Advocacy: A catch-all word for the set of skills used to create a shift in public opinion and mobilize the necessary resources and forces to support an issue, policy or constituency.

Aim: A broad statement of what will change as a result of an intervention.

Ambivalence: A conflict between two courses of action, each of which has perceived costs and benefits associated with it. The exploration and resolution of ambivalence is a key feature in motivational interviewing.

ANGELO framework: Analysis Grid for Elements [previously Environments] Linked to Obesity (Swinburn *et al.*, 1999). A standardized assessment tool for analysing environments and their impact on obesity.

Audience segmentation: Identifying who is to be targeted by an intervention according to their personal characteristics, past behaviour, and the benefits they seek.

Civil society voice: Proactive communication by the non-governmental sector (communities, NGOs, professional associations) to influence thinking and action within political space for the public good.

Cognition: Thought processes such as attention, concentration, perception, thinking, learning, memory, beliefs, expectations, and assumptions.

Cognitive behavioural therapy (CBT): A therapeutic change method addressing dysfunctional thoughts or cognitive processes and maladaptive behaviours.

Community: A group of people who have something in common. This may include living in the same geographical area or sharing common attitudes, interests or lifestyles.

Community development: An approach to development that seeks to increase the extent and effectiveness of community action, community activity, and agencies' relationships with communities.

Community mobilization: A capacity-building process through which local individuals, groups or organizations identify needs, plan, carry out and evaluate activities on a participatory and sustained basis, so as to improve health and other needs, either on their own initiative or stimulated by others.

Community participation: A process (and approach) whereby community members assume a level of responsibility and become agents for their own health and development.

Complex interventions: A broad term for any social intervention comprising multiple components.

Customer orientation: A marketing term for understanding aspects of people's lives, such as their characteristics, their needs and desires.

Evaluation: The critical assessment of the value of an activity.

Formative evaluation: An evaluation that takes place before the launch of an intervention, or during its implementation, with the goal of improving its implementation or functioning.

Group work: A method that involves the health promoter delivering to and facilitating a group, usually with a shared set of needs or characteristics.

Hard to reach: A term used used by service providers and other agencies to describe groups who experience social marginalization and stigmatization coupled with a lack of access to and engagement with health and welfare services.

Health equity: The absence of preventable health inequalities.

Health inequalities: Differences in health experience, status, and outcomes between countries, regions, and socio-economic groups.

Health-related needs: Attributes people need to have to be able to control their health-related behaviour: knowledge and awareness; access to resources; interpersonal skills and physical motor skills; and bodily autonomy.

Healthy public policy: A protocol for the common good that seeks to create a supportive environment across all areas of government jurisdiction, enabling people to live healthy lives, incorporating public accountability by government for health and health equity impact as a result of all policies enacted.

Information and advice methods: Interventions that involve the exchange of information and advice between individuals.

Intervention: Purposeful activity using finite resources that is carried out with the aim of changing something specific for a defined group of people. Sometimes the word *project* is used instead. See the explanation of terminology in the 'Overview of the book' for more on this.

Lobbying: A form of advocacy, which, through proactive and direct action, usually with remuneration or financial self-interest, applies pressure and influence on public officials and governments' formulation of policies and programs.

Mass media: Print and electronic channels through which information is transmitted to a large number of people at a time.

Method: How an intervention will achieve its aim(s), for example through the use of mass media, peer education or community mobilization.

Monitoring: The systematic collection and collation of information about the performance of an intervention or programme as it progresses. Monitoring must be based on targets set and activities agreed during the planning phases for an intervention.

Motivation: Incentives or driving forces that encourage actions: in this instance, the adoption of health-promoting behaviours of lifestyles.

Motivational interviewing: A client-centred, directive method for enhancing intrinsic motivation to change by exploring and resolving ambivalence.

Multi-level interventions: Interventions programmes that seek to address multiple levels of influence on health, such as through mixing individually focused and environmentally focused methods.

Obesogenic environment: The role environmental factors can play in determining both nutrition and physical activity.

Objectives: Specific, concrete statements of what the intervention needs to achieve in order to reach its aim.

Outcome evaluation: An evaluation that seeks to establish whether or not an intervention brought about its strategic aim.

Outreach work: A method of delivering health promotion that involves the health promoter going to a setting where the target group will be encountered, and delivering an intervention within that setting.

Participatory learning and action (PLA): PLA is a collection of methods and approaches used in action research, which enable diverse groups and individuals to learn, work, and act together in a cooperative manner, to focus on issues of joint concern, identify challenges and generate positive responses in a collaborative and democratic manner.

Peer education: An approach to health promotion that involves supporting members of a group to promote health among their peers.

Peer influence: The effects of perceptions of what peers think and do on the attitudes, values, knowledge, and behaviour of other people within their peer groups.

Peers: People who are similar to one another in terms of their age, educational or social background and experience, behaviour and/or social role.

Plan: A document produced as a result of the process of planning the intervention, which establishes the scope, aims, setting, target group, objectives, methods, and activities.

Process evaluation: A method of gathering and analysing information that helps to establish how and why an intervention brought about change.

Programme: A number of interlinked interventions (or projects) addressing a common health issue or problem (or a target group). See the explanation of terminology in the 'Overview of the book' for more on this.

Project management: The application of processes, methods, knowledge, skills, and experience to achieve the intervention or project objectives.

Public health: All organized measures to prevent disease, promote health, and prolong life among the population as a whole. See the explanation of terminology in the 'Overview of the book' for more on this.

Radio and broadcast methods: Health promotion delivered through radio or other broadcast methods such as television or internet streaming.

Settings: Physical environments with an organizational structure where people have defined roles.

Social determinants of health: Conditions that affect people's health, such as their working and living environments, income, social networks, and social position.

Social marketing: A discipline that takes the concepts of commercial marketing and applies those concepts to influence the social beliefs and behaviours of a target audience.

Social media: Media that enables interaction and exchange of information between those generating the content and those interacting with it.

Strategy: An overarching plan informed by evidence, values, and theories that sets the aims and describes how these will be achieved.

Theatre and performance methods: Health promotion delivered through performance such as dance, music, puppetry, poetry, and drama.

Transtheoretical model: Developed to describe and explain the different stages in behaviour change. The model is based on the premise that behaviour change is a process, not an event, and that individuals have different levels of motivation or readiness to change.

Young people: People in the period of transition between childhood and adulthood and therefore generally aged between 12 and 25 years old.

Index

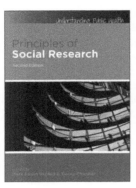

Principles of Social Research
2nd Edition

Mary Alison Durand and Tracey Chantler

ISBN: 978-0-335-26330-I (Paperback)
eBook: 978-0335-26331-8
2014

Fully updated in this second edition, this book introduces students to basic principles in social research. Taking a public health approach the book covers areas such as health promotion, public health and health services management and is aimed at helping a variety of health professionals.

Key features include:

- Extended further reading
- More indepth chapters reflecting the most current topics in the field of social research
- Increased number of international examples and updated case studies

www.openup.co.uk

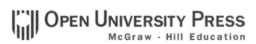

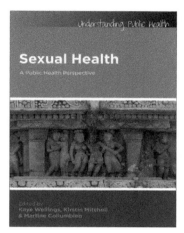

SEXUAL HEALTH
A Public Health Perspective

Kaye Wellings, Kirstin Mitchell and Martine Collumbien (Eds)

9780335244812 (Paperback)
2012

eBook also available

This timely book introduces social aspects of the study of sexual health and their application to public health practice.

The book addresses five key themes: *Conceptual and theoretical aspects of sexual health, Sexual health outcomes of risk and vulnerability, Improving sexual health status and Measuring and assessing sexual health status.* The authors consider each of these themes within their cultural and historical context and illustrate topics with international examples and case studies.

Key features:

- A spotlight on populations rather than individuals, and a focus on theprevention of ill health and promotion of well-being.
- A global perspective; the book makes the distinction between developing and developed countries, but recognises that inequalities are to be found within as well as between countries.
- A view of sexual behaviour as socially learned rather than biologically given and so as amenable to change and intervention to improve sexual health status.

www.openup.co.uk

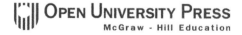

OPEN UNIVERSITY PRESS
McGraw - Hill Education

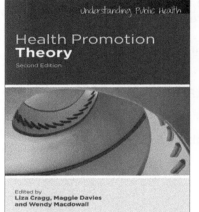

HEALTH PROMOTION THEORY
Second Edition

Liza Cragg, Maggie Davies and Wendy Macdowall

9780335263202 (Paperback)
October 2013

eBook also available

Part of the *Understanding Public Health* series, this book offers students and practitioners an accessible exploration of the origins and development of health promotion. It highlights the philosophical, ethical and political debates that influence health promotion today while also explaining the theories, frameworks and methodologies that help us understand public health problems and develop effective health promotion responses.

Key features:

- Offers more in-depth coverage of key determinants of health and how these interact with health promotion
- Revised structure to allow more depth of coverage of health promotion theory
- Updated material and case examples that reflect contemporary health promotion challenges

www.openup.co.uk

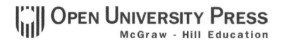

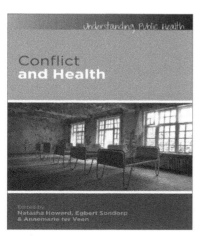

CONFLICT AND HEALTH

Natasha Howard, Egbert Sondorp and
Annemarie Ter Veen

9780335243792 (Paperback)
2012

eBook also available

Part of the popular *Understanding Public Health* series, this book provides an introductory overview of current health-related challenges and policy debates on appropriate responses to different humanitarian conflicts. Written by experts, it explores the context of conflict and health, the interventions used in humanitarian crises and post-conflict resolution issues.

Key features:

- Uses case studies and real examples to highlight best practice in healthcare provision
- Written from an international perspective
- Considers post-conflict resolution issues

www.openup.co.uk

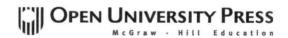

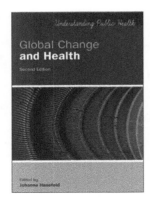

Globalization and Health
2nd Edition

Johanna Hanefeld

ISBN: 978-0-335-26408-7 (Paperback)
eBook: 978-0-335-26409-4
2015

Global health is a relatively new but rapidly expanding field as public health practitioners recognize the important challenges that global changes are posing for human health. Health issues are increasingly crossing national boundaries, and this book explores the actors that shape global health and explores some of the key issues in global health.

Key topics include:

- Social change linked to globalization
- Governance of global health
- Pharmaceuticals and tobacco

www.openup.co.uk

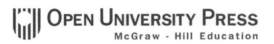

OPEN UNIVERSITY PRESS
McGraw - Hill Education